Comprehensive Maxillofacial Osteomyelitis

Authored by

Deepak Gupta

Soheyl Sheikh

&

Shambulingappa Pallagatti

Department of Oral Medicine and Radiology, M.M. College of Dental Sciences and Research, Mullana, Ambala, Haryana, India

General:

1. Any dispute or claim arising out of or in connection with this License Agreement or the Work (including non-contractual disputes or claims) will be governed by and construed in accordance with the laws of the U.A.E. as applied in the Emirate of Dubai. Each party agrees that the courts of the Emirate of Dubai shall have exclusive jurisdiction to settle any dispute or claim arising out of or in connection with this License Agreement or the Work (including non-contractual disputes or claims).
2. Your rights under this License Agreement will automatically terminate without notice and without the need for a court order if at any point you breach any terms of this License Agreement. In no event will any delay or failure by Bentham Science Publishers in enforcing your compliance with this License Agreement constitute a waiver of any of its rights.
3. You acknowledge that you have read this License Agreement, and agree to be bound by its terms and conditions. To the extent that any other terms and conditions presented on any website of Bentham Science Publishers conflict with, or are inconsistent with, the terms and conditions set out in this License Agreement, you acknowledge that the terms and conditions set out in this License Agreement shall prevail.

Bentham Science Publishers Ltd.
Executive Suite Y - 2
PO Box 7917, Saif Zone
Sharjah, U.A.E.
Email: subscriptions@benthamscience.org

BENTHAM SCIENCE

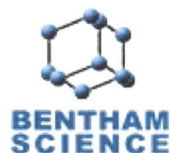

CONTENTS

FOREWORD

It is my honor and pleasure to write this foreword for Dr. Deepak Gupta's book on osteomyelitis of the jaw bones. It takes a lot of time to make a decision to write a text book for clinicians and it takes even more efforts and energy to finish it.

The topic of this text book is well chosen and well considered and contributes to the dental and medical profession. Even in the era of abundant use of antibiotics, osteomyelitis is still an issue, which can lead to debilitating and disfiguring lesions in the maxillofacial region, as early diagnosis is a key. With patients and doctors being more mobile and moving to different parts of the world, it is important now that the doctors recognize the pathology, which they may have never seen in their home country.

The information and expert material in this book are paramount for dental clinicians as this manuscript contains crucial information about the pathology, aetiology and the therapy or treatment approach for patients with osteomyelitis lesions. Information about which diagnostic imaging modalities can and should be used is also nicely illustrated and backed up with qualitative literature.

I am convinced that this book will find its place in many dental offices, clinics and universities.

I congratulate Dr. Deepak Gupta for his formidable work.

Johan Aps
Dentomaxillofacial Radiology
University of Western Australia, Dental School
Australia

PREFACE

The word osteomyelitis is made up of a combination of two or three small words. In the Greek terminology, the word **"OSTEON"** means bone, the word "**MYELOS**" means marrow, and **"ITIS"** means inflammation. Henceforth, osteomyelitis may be considered as an inflammatory condition of the bone that usually begins as an infection of the medullary cavity, rapidly involves harversian systems and quickly extends to the periosteum area. It is considered to be a bacterial disease and was believed to be caused primarily by *Staphylococcus aureus*, Staphylococcus epidermidis, or hemolytic streptococci. But in recent years it has been found that 93% percent of the osteomyelitic infections of the jaws are polymicrobial with an average of 3.9 organisms per specimen. The most common predisposing factors for osteomyelitis to occur include irradiation, immunosuppressant treatment, malnutrition, and metabolic bone disease. It can also be precipitated by Paget's disease of bone, fibrous dysplasia and bone tumors.

Osteomyelitis disease can involve any bone of the body. Bones of the jaws are also prone to develop this disease. Earlier before the advent of antibiotics, osteomyelitis of the jaws was frequently encountered as a result of odontogenic infections and was considered fatal. But with the advent of pertinent antibiotics, it was possible to control this disease. Literature reveals that the mandible is more commonly affected than the maxilla since the mandible is poorly vascularized as compared to the maxilla. The most common cause of osteomyelitis (OM) of the jaws is the spread of adjacent odontogenic infection. The second most common cause is the osteomyelitis occurring after a maxillofacial fracture, usually of the mandible.

The signs and symptoms of different types of osteomyelitis of jaws may include pain, which may be severe, throbbing and deep seated during initial stages. Later it may also lead to swelling, trismus, suppuration, fistula formation and fetid odour. It may further result in fibromyalgia, dysphagia, cervical lymphadenitis, paresthesia, fever, malaise and anorexia. Clinically pus exudation may be seen from around the neck of the teeth or from an extraction socket or from other sites. It starts as acute osteomyelitis. If the infection is not controlled, the process becomes chronic. This may even lead to loosening of teeth as well as sequestra formation. Untreated chronic osteomyelitis may even lead to pathological fracture.

Diagnostic imaging of osteomyelitis has been performed primarily through conventional radiographic modalities. These include intraoral periapical radiography, occlusal radiography and panoramic radiography. Advanced imaging modalities include computed tomography, magnetic resonance imaging (MRI) and bone scintigraphy. Since Maxillofacial osteomyelitis is chronic and debilitating disease, the main aim of the dental professionals is to diagnose the disease at early stages so as to initiate prompt treatment. Henceforth, there must be regular dental assessment and care.

ACKNOWLEDGEMENTS

For this Book my sincere thanks first of all goes to the Almighty, who brought me on this stage to meet my long cherished desire. In fact, it would have been impossible without His hidden unprecedented help and grace. I wish to express my sincere gratitude towards my guide, supervisor and teachers whom I would like to emulate.

I express my whole hearted and humble thanks to my beloved parents **Mrs. Sunita Gupta &** **Mr. Ravinder Kumar Gupta** whose unforgettable sacrifices and choicest blessings provided me the opportunity to be educated. My deep sense of obligation to them will ever remain for their constant inspiration and encouragement throughout the course of this task.

I am thankful to my wife **Dr. Sonam Gupta**, who showed her fervent interest, unusual generosity, accommodative attitude and gave me invaluable love, care and affection to accomplish this work.

I extend deep sense of gratitude to my brother **Dr. Maqul Gupta and his wife Mrs. Mini Gupta** for their unflinching moral support. They took personal interest and gave me constant encouragement since the inception of this work.

I owe gratitude to my mentors **Dr. Amit Mittal** (Vice-Principal, MMIMSR, Mullana) and **Dr. Sanjeev Gupta** (Professor and Head, Dept. of Dermatology, MMIMSR, Mullana) for their richness of vast experience and invaluable support throughout my academic carrier.

I would also like to thank my colleagues **Dr. Amit Aggarwal, Dr. Ravinder Singh, Dr. Preeti Garg, Dr. Rahul Bansal, Dr. Johan Aps** and **Dr. Ibrahim Nasseh** for their invaluable support and help throughout the process of completion of this task.

A special thanks to **Dr. Debdutta Das** (Principal, MMCDSR, Mullana) and **Dr. Monika Das** for their inspiring attitude and richness of vast experience.

CONFLICT OF INTEREST

There is no conflict of interest regarding publication of this book.

Deepak Gupta
Department of Oral Medicine and Radiology,
M.M. College of Dental Sciences and Research,
Mullana, Ambala, Haryana,
India
E-mail: drdeepak_26@rediffmail.com

List of Facilitators

Aps Johan K	Department of Pediatric Dentistry, Director of ORIS (Oral Radiology Interpretation Service), University of Washington, Associate Editor of Dentomaxillofacial Radiology (BIR Journal)
Nasseh Ibrahim	Oral Medicine and Maxillofacial Radiologist,
Mittal Amit	Dept of Radiodiagnosis and Imaging, MMIMSR, M.M. University, Mullana,
Gupta Sanjeev	Dept of Dermatology, MMIMSR, M.M. University, Mullana,
Gupta Sonam	Private Practitioner, Dental Surgeon,
Aggarwal Amit	Dept of Oral Medicine and Radiology, MMCDSR, Mullana,
Singh Ravinder	Dept of Oral Medicine and Radiology, MMCDSR, Mullana,
Garg Preeti	Dept of Oral Medicine and Radiology, MMCDSR, Mullana,
Bansal Rahul	Dept of Oral Medicine and Radiology, MMCDSR, Mullana,
Gupta Maqul	General Physician, Enlive health,

CHAPTER 1

Introduction

Abstract: Osteomyelitis of the jaws is a challenging disease for the clinicians and the patients despite many advances in the diagnosis and treatment. It was a common and dreaded disease in the past because of its prolonged course and uncertainty of outcome. It is an interesting fact to know that the oral cavity is among the most biologically dynamic tissues of human body. Any adverse change arising from any immunosuppressive systemic disease will readily manifest itself in the oral cavity. Osteomyelitis is not an exception to this. Thus, a careful evaluation of an apparently healthy individual presenting with a jaw swelling that may be associated with odontogenic infection must always be emphasized. This particular chapter will provide a brief introduction to the Osteomyelitis of the jaws so as to orient the readers towards the disease, its etiopathogenesis and clinicopathological features.

Keywords: Etiopathogenesis, Inflammation, Mandible, Maxilla, Osteomyelitis of the jaws.

Osteomyelitis is an inflammation of the medullary portion of the bone. It usually also affects the cortical bone and periosteum. The process is rarely confined to the endosteum. Therefore osteomyelitis may be considered as an inflammatory condition of the bone that usually begins as an infection of the medullary cavity, rapidly involves harversian systems and quickly extends to the periosteum area [1].

The word osteomyelitis is made up of a combination of two or three small words. The word **"OSSEOUS"** in Latin means bony, while **"OSTEON"** in Greek means bone. **"MYELOS"** in Greek means marrow; and **"ITIS"** in Greek means inflammation [2].

In the past, osteomyelitis of jaws like that of long bones was believed to be caused primarily by *Staphylococcus aureus*, Staphylococcus epidermidis, or hemolytic streptococci. But in recent years, several anaerobic bacteria have been identified thus adding to the number of microbiologic agents involved in the disease [1]. It has been found that 93% percent of the osteomyelitic infections of the jaws are polymicrobial with an average of 3.9 organisms per specimen [1].

The most common and possible predisposing factors that should be considered for osteomyelitis to occur include irradiation, immunosuppressant treatment, malnutrition, and metabolic bone disease [2]. It can also be precipitated by Paget's disease of bone, fibrous dysplasia and bone tumors [3].

Infection with human immunodeficiency virus must also be considered as a precipitating factor to osteomyelitis as it diminishes body's natural defense mechanisms [3].

Osteomyelitis of the jaws is associated with different etiologic hypothesis. However, the circulation of the affected area as well as the patient's immune response is likely to be of the utmost importance [4].

It is more common in men as compared to women. Incidence of osteomyelitis is less in the maxillary bone as compared to mandible because the maxillary bone has got a better blood supply, thin cortical plates and there is relative paucity of medullary tissue which precludes confinement of infection within the bone and permits dissipation of edema. On the contrary, infantile osteomyelitis is more common in the maxilla than the mandible as it spreads by hematogenous route.

The portal of entry of the offensive microorganisms may have most likely been through the inflamed periodontal tissues while a haematogenous spread of the microbes may be contemplated in an immunosuppressed state [3].

Osteomyelitis has a range of clinical presentations depending on the virulence of the infecting organisms, the resistance of the host, and the reaction of the bone and periosteum to the inflammation.

Historically osteomyelitis was a frequently encountered infection in dental practice. Osteomyelitis of jaws is becoming much less common nowadays [1, 2].This is attributed to improved nutrition, the availability of antibiotic therapy as well as early diagnosis and early therapeutic intervention due to new imaging modalities [1].

Advances in the fields of anesthesia, antibiotic therapy, preventive and restorative dentistry as well as the availability of competent medical and dental care have reduced the incidence of the disease dramatically. However when osteomyelitis does occur in contemporary dental practice, its management is often associated with substantial morbidity due to the natural course of the disease and the consequences of its treatment.

However on the contrary, osteomyelitis of the jaws may happen as a consequence of dental treatment too. In other words even a healthy individual can develop osteomyelitis of the jaws as a consequence of root canal therapy.

Acute osteomyelitis may progress to subacute or chronic stage if the treatment has been inadequate or if there is delay in the diagnosis of the condition. It is estimated that 30% of osteomyelitis infections become chronic. Therefore, early diagnosis and adequate treatment of acute osteomyelitis is crucial.

It can lead to occasional disfigurement and dysfunction of the concerned maxillofacial area resulting from the loss of teeth and bones and accompanied facial scarring. The keystones leading to the diagnosis of this condition are characteristic but not pathognomonic [5].

Diagnostic imaging of osteomyelitis has been performed primarily through conventional radiographic modalities. These include intraoral periapical radiography, occlusal radiography and panoramic radiography. Advanced imaging modalities include computed tomography, magnetic resonance imaging (MRI) and bone scintigraphy [6].

To further complicate matters, multidrug resistance has also contributed to longer treatment times, increased morbidity and death. Bacterial tolerance to antibiotics is poorly understood and often negatively affects treatment outcomes. Henceforth new directions in oral surgery, orthopedics, infectious diseases, immunology, and radiology are required that may have the application to the treatment of maxillofacial osteomyelitis.

In this book, an attempt has been made to understand the nature of osteomyelitis, its etiopathogenesis, clinicopathological features and diagnostic criteria. It is emphasized that early diagnosis is a key-factor to reduce morbidity and initiate prompt early management.

CHAPTER 2

History, Epidemiology and Incidence

Abstract: This particular chapter highlights how medical profession over the years has evolved regarding the concept of osteomyelitis of the jaws. Before the antibiotic era, it was considered as a dreaded disease. Nowadays, with the advent of antibiotics, osteomyelitis can be easily controlled. The dental science has succeeded to the heights that it is even not common for people to develop osteomyelitis often as compared to the incidence of osteomyelitis in the past. The patients opt for timely as well as better dental treatment modalities. Furthermore, dental professionals perform the dental treatment taking care of the systemic condition of the patient too. This has reduced the occurrence of osteomyelitis of the jaws. As far as the Epidemiology is concerned, Osteomyelitis of jaws is uncommon in developed countries, but it continues to be a source of significant concern in developing nations.

Keywords: Epidemiology of Osteomyelitis of jaws, Homo erectus, Incidence of Osteomyelitis of jaws, Odontogenic infection, Osteomyelitis of the jaws, Sequestra, Turkana Boy.

History

Osteomyelitis can be considered as one of the oldest diseases known to affect human beings [7]. The term Osteomyelitis was first coined by **Nelaton** in **1844**.

Osteomyelitis of the jaws is a disease that has affected mankind since prehistory. This can be well documented by the famous 1.6 million-year old fossil find of "Turkana Boy". This fossil is of a 12-year-old prehuman hominid (homo erectus). His nearly complete skeleton was found which clearly showed osteomyelitis arising around one of his first molar teeth due to an odontogenic infection. Paleontologists even stress that osteomyelitis was the most likely cause of his premature death [8].

It was a frequently encountered infection in the dental practice in the past but the incidence of this disease has reduced to a great extent nowadays. This fact is further supported by isolated case reports of this disease in the literature in the last few decades.

Mowlem in **1945** implicated paradoxical tooth extraction as an etiological factor for osteomyelitis [9]. This condition has been reported a number of times in infants [9].

Rees was the first to refer this disease in infants in **1847 [9]**.

Wass in **1948** has paid emphasis on the role of anaemia in producing diminished resistance to osteomyelitis of the mandible [9].

Osteomyelitis of the jaws is well documented in the standard texts like **Killey** and **Kay** in **1970** and **Shafer** *et al.* in **1974 [9]**. It was **Killey** *et al.* in **1971** who stated that osteomyelitis is rare in maxilla due to excellent blood supply.

With the passage of time, the prevalence, clinical course as well as the management of osteomyelitis of the jawbones has changed. These changes have taken place over the past 50 years. This is attributed to advances in the fields of anaesthesia, antibiotic therapy, preventive and restorative dentistry. The availability of competent medical and dental care has also added on to the above said changes in the disease [7].

In the preantibiotic era, **Wassmund** in **1935** and **Axhausen** in **1934** stated that the jaw bone osteomyelitis can be classically represented as an acute onset osteomyelitis. This was usually followed by transition to a secondary chronic process later on. The clinical symptoms of this disease included widespread bone necroses, neo-osteogenesis, large sequester formation, and intra and extra oral fistula formation. These presentations, sometimes lead to significant facial disfigurement [8].

The treatment of osteomyelitis of jaw bones was also well established and was practiced in the past. The role of antibiotic therapy for resolution of the disease was stated by **Walker** in **1947**. He stressed upon the early as well as adequate antibiotic therapy for the disease [9].

Until the mid-twentieth century, the treatment of osteomyelitis of the jaws, like osteomyelitis of long bones in other parts of the skeleton had been primarily surgical. Back then, osteomyelitis of the jaws was an infectious disease with an often complicated course, involving multiple surgical interventions and usually leading to facial disfigurement as a result of loss of affected bone and teeth and the accompanying scarring. However, since the second half of the past century there has been a dramatic reduction of the incidence of osteomyelitis cases involving the jaws and other bones of the skeleton as advocated by **Hudson** in **1993**. The major responsible factor leading to this development must probably be seen in the introduction of antibiotics to the therapeutic armamentarium.

However, improved nutrition, and better availability to medical and dental care, especially including advances in preventive dentistry and oral hygiene have also contributed well to the above said fact [8].

Archer in **1975** advocated that hospitalization should be considered in the patients suffering from osteomyelitis. Further, the administration of loads of penicillin for the same was stressed upon. He also advised rest for the affected patients along with good dietary intake [9]. After the introduction of antibiotics, acute phases were often concealed by these antimicrobial drugs without fully eliminating the infection. Sub-acute or chronic forms of osteomyelitis have therefore become more prominent without an actual acute phase [8].

Epidemiology and Incidence

Nowadays osteomyelitis is a rare disease in developed countries of **Europe and North America** [9]. Over the past 25 years, clinical reports on osteomyelitis have been found to be infrequent in medical literature but with several exceptions[7].

Adekeye *et al.* in **1975**, **Adekeye & Shamia** in **1976** and **Daramola & Ajagbe** in **1982** carried out studies on **Nigerian population** and concluded that the classic osteomyelitis presenting with multiple sinuses, massive sequestration and eventual ankylosis was not uncommon at that time [9]. Apart from a few reviews from Nigeria, only isolated case reports can be found in the literature of the last 3 decades [9].

Osteomyelitis was prevalent in **African** population in **1980's** and it posed a major surgical problem at that time [10].

The review done by **Daramola &Ajagbe** in **1982** and **Adekeye & Cornah** in **1985** of large series from **Nigerian population** revealed that the commonest aetiological factor for osteomyelitis was periodontal disease [10].

Adekeye *et al.* in **1975** in **Nigeria** showed that there are certain factors which contributed to cases of pyogenic osteomyelitis of mandible and maxilla in Nigerian children. Such factors were malnutrition, malaria, anaemia and acute eruptive fevers particularly measles [9].

Kinman and Lee in **1968** studied cases of chronic osteomyelitis in **Singapore**. They concluded that most cases of chronic osteomyelitis of the mandible were found to develop in undernourished individuals [9].

Masahiko *et al.* in **1987** stressed that osteomyelitis is a common inflammatory condition among inflammatory diseases of jawbones and is usually seen in adults [11].

McCash *et al.* in **1953** contributed to the fact that it is relatively rare in children although it is well known in newborn infants [12].

True progressive Osteomyelitis of jaws is uncommon in developed countries, but it continues to be a source of significant concern in developing nations. In Europe and North America, most cases arise after odontogenic infections or traumatic fracture of the jaws. In Africa many cases reported occur in the presence of ANUG (Acute Necrotizing Ulcerative Gingivitis) or NOMA [13].

The overall incidence internationally is higher in developing countries [4] while in the US the overall prevalence is 1 per 5,000 children. Neonatal prevalence is approximately 1 per 1,000. The annual incidence in sickle cell patients is approximately 0.36%. The prevalence of Osteomyelitis after foot puncture may be as high as 16%. The prevalence increases up to 30-40% in patients with diabetes [14].

Male-to-female ratio is approximately 2:1 and it has a bimodal age distribution [14].

Morbidity can be significant. The sequelae can include localized spread of infection to associated soft tissues or joints, progression to chronic infection with pain and disability, generalized infection, or sepsis. In severe cases amputation of the involved extremity may be required. **Aslangul** *et al.* in **2005** revealed that up to 10-15% of patients with vertebral osteomyelitis will develop neurologic findings or frank spinal-cord compression [14].

Mortality rates are low, unless associated sepsis or an underlying serious medical condition is present [14].

CHAPTER 3

Etiology and Pathogenesis

Abstract: Osteomyelitis of jaws is a multifactorial disease. It has various etiological factors which lead to the inflammation of the medullary portion of the bone. The various predisposing factors for osteomyelitis include immunosuppressive conditions, malnutrition, metabolic bone disease, tobacco, alcohol, odontogenic infections, *etc*. Sometimes haematogenous dissemination of infection to healthy bones and infection associated with peripheral vascular disease may also lead to maxillofacial osteomyelitis. The process leading to osteomyelitis is initiated by acute inflammation which leads to hyperaemia, increased capillary permeability and infiltration of leukocytes which further results in destruction of bacteria and vascular thrombosis. The process also leads to release of proteolytic enzymes which causes tissue necrosis and accumulation of pus. This results in the rise of intramedullary pressure resulting in vascular collapse, venous stasis and ischemia of the concerned area. The pus then travels through the haversian and nutrient canals and accumulates beneath the periosteum of the bone leading to its elevation from the underlying cortex which further reduces the vascular supply to the bone. This is vascular impairment in the jaw which is a contributory factor in the development of osteomyelitis.

Keywords: Haversian and nutrient canals, Hyperaemia, Intramedullary pressure, Odontogenic infections, Osteomyelitis of jaws, Periosteum, Vascular thrombosis.

Etiology

Koorbusch & Fotos in 1992 and Asseri *et al.* in 1997 commented on the predisposing factors that should be considered for osteomyelitis to occur. These include irradiation, immunosuppressive conditions, malnutrition and metabolic bone disease [7]. It can also be precipitated by Paget's disease of bone, fibrous dysplasia and bone tumors [3].

Khosla and Rosenfield in 1971 implicated tobacco, drugs and alcohol along with diabetes, malignancy, malnutrition, osteoporosis, anaemia and AIDS as the predisposing factors for osteomyelitis [7, 15].

Apart from this, **Koorbusch, Fotos and Goll in 1992** found hypertension, pulmonary disease, immunosuppression, rheumatoid arthritis, hepatitis, hypothyroidism, recurrent pneumonia, and toxic chemical exposure associated with the incidence of maxillofacial osteomyelitis [7].

Pantaleo *et al.* **in 1993** advocated that the infection with human immunodeficiency virus is a precipitating factor for osteomyelitis as it diminishes the body's natural defence mechanisms [3].

Adekeye and Cornah in 1985 highlighted six possible etiological factors for osteomyelitis of the jaws. They comprise odontogenic infections, cancrum oris, tooth extraction, acute ulcerative gingivitis, fractures and periodontal disease in descending order of prevalence [9].

Adekeye *et al.* **in 1975** and **Adekeye & Cornah in 1985** advocated that the contribution of odontogenic infections and ulcerative gingivitis to osteomyelitis in the maxilla were almost equal to that of cancrum oris. However, in mandible, odontogenic infections, periodontal disease, and tooth extraction played a far greater role in the etiology than cancrum oris [9].

This was further confirmed by **Lawoyin** *et al.* **in 1988** as he found periodontal disease associated with lower left molar teeth as a causative factor for osteomyelitis of mandible. Osteomyelitis was also found arising *de novo* in the malar bone without any possible causative factor identified. Hematogenous spread was the possible explanation but there was lack of any evidence [9].

Koorbusch, Fotos and Goll in 1992 considered the contiguous spread of odontogenic infections as the primary [7] and the most common aetiological factor of the disease [1]. They stated that these infections originate from pulpal or periodontal tissues, pericoronitis, infected socket or infected cyst [1, 16].

According to **Koorbusch, Fotos and Goll in 1992,** various forms of trauma, especially compound fractures were the second leading cause of jaw osteomyelitis [7]. Other causes of the infection were neoplasia and radiation. It can also occur following infection at the areas where surgery is done [16]. Additional trauma to a pre-existing chronic local infection carries a great risk of causing deep bone infection. Foreign bodies as well as the various transplants and implants used in maxillofacial and dental surgery may also harbour microorganisms and hence facilitate further spread to the surrounding bone [8].

A relatively small number of jaw infections also occur secondary to periostitis caused by gingival ulceration [1]. Lastly, osteomyelitis can also be initiated by a contiguous focus of infection or hematogenous spread in a very infrequent number [1]. This may include spread of infection by furuncle on the face, wound on the skin, upper respiratory tract infections, middle ear infections or mastoiditis [1].

Steiner *et al.* in 1983 stated that haematogenous dissemination of infection to healthy bones and infection associated with peripheral vascular disease were other causes of maxillofacial osteomyelitis apart from Odontogenic infections [10].

Systemic tuberculosis can also serve as an etiological factor for osteomyelitis of the jaws. **Chaudhary, Kalra and Gomber in 2004** stated that tuberculous osteomyelitis is very rare and constitutes less than 2% of the skeletal tuberculosis. Jaw involvement in TB is very rare and usually affects older individuals [17].

Soman & Davis in 2003 and **Dinkar & Prabhudesai in 2008** advocated that about half of such patients do not have pulmonary disease at the time they report as the primary infection heals leaving some surviving tubercle bacilli [18].With lowering of resistance, these are reactivated producing local as well as heamatogenous spread [18, 19].

Johnston *et al.* in 1968 and **Steiner *et al.* in 1983** stated that the osteomyelitis is a well recognized hazard in osteoporosis due to reduced blood circulation to the bone as a result of obliteration and fibrosis of the bone marrow [10].

Although there are several etiological factors, acute and secondary chronic osteomyelitis represents a true infection of the bone induced by pyogenic microorganisms [8]. A single pathogenic species always recovered from the lesion is Staphylococcus species [1]. This is supported by the reviews on **Nigerian population** done by **Daramola & Ajagbe in 1982** and **Adekeye & Cornah in 1985** that have shown *Staphylococcus aureus* to be the most common organism recovered from such lesions.

Pathogenesis

As stated earlier, osteomyelitis (Fig. **3.1**) is caused by contiguous focus of infection or haematogenous spread [1, 7, 9, 15]. The process leading to osteomyelitis is initiated by acute inflammation which leads to hyperaemia and increased capillary permeability. This process will also be accompanied by infiltration of leukocytes as described by **Koorbusch and Fotos in 1992** [7]. As destruction of bacteria and vascular thrombosis is produced, there is release of proteolytic enzymes which causes tissue necrosis [1, 16].

Due to accumulation of pus (Fig. **3.2**), the intramedullary pressure raises resulting in vascular collapse and venous stasis. This pus is composed of necrotic tissue, dead bacteria and white blood cells. This will further lead to ischemia of the concerned area [16].

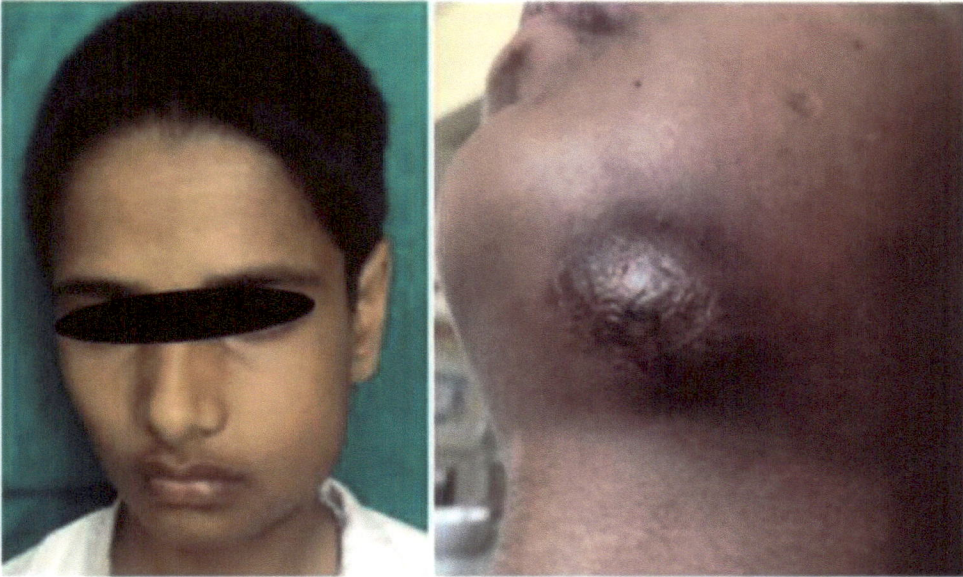

Fig. (3.1). Extraoral profile of the patient with swelling on the left side of the face. Evidence of extraoral sinus in the parasymphyseal region.

The pus then travels through the haversian and nutrient canals and accumulates beneath the periosteum of the bone leading to its elevation from the underlying cortex. This will further reduce the vascular supply to the bone (Fig. **3.2**). **Wannfors and Gazelius in 1991** stated that vascular impairment in the jaw could be a contributory factor in the development of osteomyelitic disease [20].Compression of neurovascular bundle accelerates thrombosis and ischemia and results in inferior alveolar nerve dysfunction.

This elevation of the periosteum from the underlying cortex depends upon its attachment to the bone. Greater the elevation, more is the ischemia produced. Extensive periosteal elevation occurs more frequently in children as compared to adults. This is because the periosteum is bound less firmly to bone in children than in adults.

The periosteum is penetrated by the pus in later stages if pus continues to accumulate. This will present as mucosal and cutaneous abscess and fistulas may also develop (Fig. **3.1**).

The osteomyelitic process may become chronic as the effectiveness of the host defence system as well as the therapy increases. At this stage, the inflammation is regressed and formation of granulation tissue takes place. Also there is formation of new blood vessels which lyse the bone. This leads to separation of fragments of necrotic bone from the viable bone. These fragments are known as *sequestra* [1].

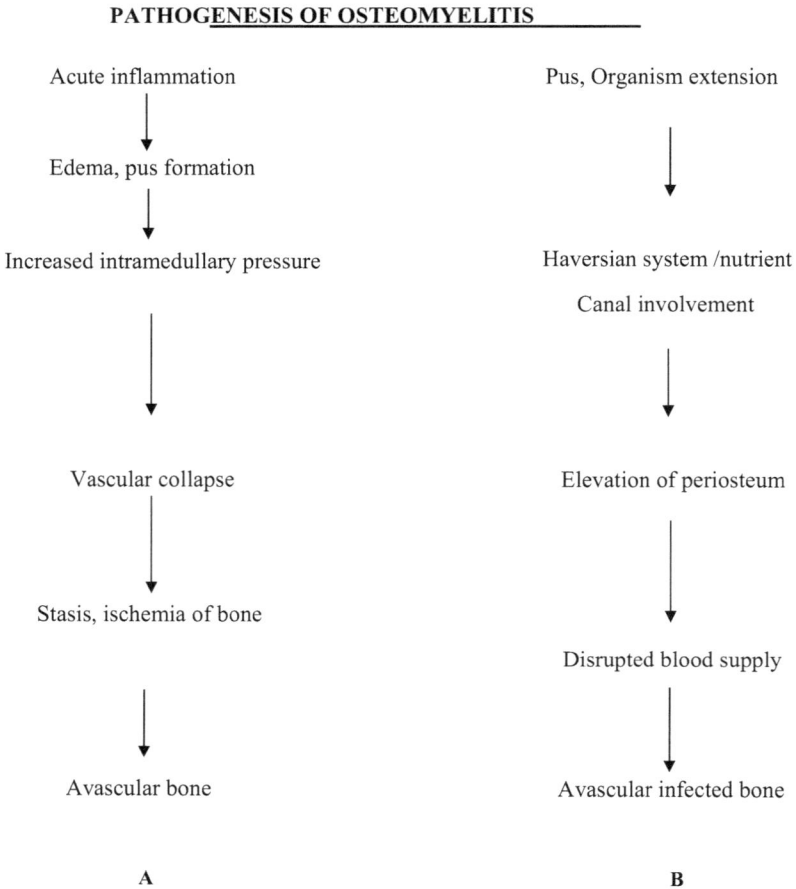

PATHOGENESIS OF OSTEOMYELITIS

Acute inflammation   Pus, Organism extension

↓   ↓

Edema, pus formation

↓

Increased intramedullary pressure   Haversian system /nutrient

Canal involvement

↓   ↓

Vascular collapse   Elevation of periosteum

↓   ↓

Stasis, ischemia of bone

Disrupted blood supply

↓   ↓

Avascular bone   Avascular infected bone

A   B

A. Inflammation leading to avascular bone.

B. Extension of pus & microorganisms.

Fig. (3.2). Pathogenesis of osteomyelitis [1].

Adekeye and Cornah in 1985 found that sequestrum formation is an inevitable consequence of established osteomyelitis and is found in 90% of the maxillary and in 75% of the mandibular cases. This higher incidence of sequestration in maxilla is attributed to greater prevalence of cancrum oris and acute ulcerative gingivitis in the aetiology of maxillary osteomyelitis [9]. Occasionally a hemimandible or a whole of mandible can convert into a sequestrum [9].

Small sections of bone may be lysed completely, whereas larger ones may be isolated by a bed of granulation tissue encased in a sheath of new bone known as involucrum [1].

Bone surrounding a sequestrum sometimes appears radiographically as less densely mineralized than the sequestrum itself because increased vascularity of adjacent vital bone creates a relative demineralization [1]. In other words, this devitalized island of cortical bone *i.e. sequestrum,* becomes favourable for precipitation of ionized calcium which is mobilized by surrounding osteolytic process [16].

The sequestra may get revascularized, remain quiescent, resorb, or can be infected chronically. According to **Adekeye and Cornah in 1985,** sequestra requires surgical removal before the infection subsides completely [9]. Occasionally the involucrum is penetrated by cloacae *i.e.* vascular channels through which pus escapes to an epithelial surface.

Osteomyelitis of the Jaws

Osteomyelitis of the jaws is relatively less frequent as compared to that of long bones. One of the most important factors in the establishment of osteomyelitis is compromised blood supply of the particular region.

Osteomyelitis in the Maxilla

Osteomyelitis in the maxilla occurs much less frequently than that of the mandible because the blood supply in case of maxilla is more extensive as compared to the mandible, a view supported by **Killey *et al.* in 1971.**

Mowlem in 1945 pointed that the vascular anatomy of the maxilla consists of a series of vascular arcades with free anastomoses thus producing generous blood supply [9]. Radiographic support for this view was produced by **Bradley in 1975** who studied carotid angiograms of the maxilla from a series of patients and cadavers and demonstrated a good network of vessels in contradistinction to the mandible where the inferior alveolar artery was found frequently occluded in subjects over 40 years of age [9].

Moreover, the presence of thin cortical plates and a relative paucity of medullary tissues in the maxilla preclude confinement of infections within the bone. This will permit the dissipation of edema and pus into the soft tissues and the paranasal sinuses.

On the contrary, **Adekeye and Cornah in 1985** advocated that infantile osteomyelitis is more common in the maxilla than the mandible as it spreads by hematogenous route [9]. This is because the maxilla being more vascular, the chances of the lesion occurring in infants is raised. Hematogenous origin of the disease and predisposition from local trauma to alveolar mucosa either at or shortly after birth were considered in the pathogenesis of acute maxillary osteomyelitis in infancy by **Wilensky in 1932 [9]**.

Further **Asherson in 1939 and Haward & Robinson in 1948** considered the role of staphylococcal infection of first deciduous molar tooth bud in the pathogenesis of osteomyelitis of jaws.

Macbeth in 1951 considered infection of the maxillary antrum in the pathogenesis of infantile osteomyelitis of the jaws [9].

Osteomyelitis in the Mandible

The mandible resembles long bones as it has a medullary cavity, dense cortical plates, and a well defined periosteum. Bone marrow is composed of sinusoids rich in reticuloendothelial cells, erythrocytes, granulocytes, platelets, oeteoblastic precursors, cancellous bone, fat and blood vessels. The marrow space is lined by the endosteum, a membrane of cells containing large number of osteoblasts. Bone spicules radiate centrally from cortical bone to produce a scaffold of interconnecting trabeculae.The distinctive architecture of cortical bone includes longitudinally oriented haversian systems known as osteons, each with a central canal and a blood vessel that provides nutrients by means of canaliculi to osteocytes.

Except for the coronoid process, which is supplied by temporalis muscle vessels, the mandible receives its blood supply from the inferior alveolar artery as reviewed by **Wannfors and Gazelius in 1991 [20]**.

A secondary source is the periosteal supply, which generally runs parallel to the cortical surface of the bone, giving off nutrient vessels that penetrate the cortical bone and anastomose with the branches of the inferior alveolar artery [16]. Mandibular venous drainage proceeds upward to the pharyngeal plexus through the inferior dental veins and downward to the external jugular veins [16].

Waldron in 1943 gave an exhaustive description of vascular morphology of the mandible and associated structures to account for the spread of osteomyelitis. He described mandibular vascular support as being provided through multiple arterial loops from a single major vessel, which renders large portion of bone susceptible to necrosis with the occurrence of major vessel infectious thrombosis [16].

Waldervogel in 1970 described the relationship of osteomyelitis to vascular support of long bones of developing and adult human skeleton. He made several conclusions [16]:

   i. There tend to be segregation of vascular channels, which act like "end organs", due to lack of terminal collateral anastomosis, ultimately leading to vascular plugging by bacteria, microthrombi or both.
  ii. When afferent vessels anastomose with medullary channels, there is a possibility of a decrease in venous flow with associated areas of greater turbulence.
iii. There may be a reduction in host immune defense mechanisms associated with these vascular channels in calcified tissues [16].

CHAPTER 4

Classification

Abstract: The classification of a disease is considered as a mandatory step so as to properly understand its various presentations. This also aids to formulate a favourable management plan best suited for the patient. Attributing to this fact, various researchers have proposed different classification systems of osteomyelitis in the literature. These different classification systems are based on Anatomic position, Clinical presentation, Pathological features or Radiological features of the disease. Some of the authors have even classified osteomyelitis on the basis of etiology and pathogenesis too. Henceforth there are multiple classification systems of osteomyelitis of the jaws throughout the literature. Authors also believe that these multiple classification systems has created confusion and hindered the comparative studies for the same. This in turn affects the pertinent management. This particular chapter highlights various classification systems of osteomyelitis of jaws.

Keywords: Acute Osteomyelitis, Chronic Osteomyelitis, Classification of Osteomyelitis of jaws, Non-suppurative osteomyelitis, Suppurative Osteomyelitis, Zurich Classification of Osteomyelitis.

The clinicians and the students may wonder as to why all the diseases have their classification system. Further it is also evident that the diseases may also possess multiple types of classification systems. This may be attributed to the fact that the classification system helps to pertinently access the severity or treatment planning of that particular disease. Similarly, the literature reveals wide variety of classification systems for Osteomyelitis of jaws. These classifications were based upon the aetiology, pathogenesis, anatomy or physiology of the bone.

Following is the Overview of Currently Used Classification Systems for osteomyelitis.

A) Waldvogel and Medoff in 1970 were the first ones to provide a widely accepted staging system for osteomyelitis of long bones. They classified osteomyelitis into three categories on the basis of etiopathogenesis of the disease [8]. It includes the following classification:

Deepak Gupta, Soheyl Skeikh & Shambulingappa Pallagatti

a) *According to duration*: Acute or Chronic

b) *According to source of infection*: Osteomyelitis from haematogenous spread due to bacteraemia or from a contiguous focus *i.e.* infection of any nearby tissue.

c) *Osteomyelitis due to vascular insufficiency.*

Drawback: It doesn't explain the infection of bone due to direct penetration of the microorganism during trauma or during surgery [8]. Literature highlights that this classification system does not help the clinician to frame therapeutic strategies for osteomyelitis that whether the disease will be managed surgically or with antibiotic therapy [8].

B) Cierny *et al.* in 1985 and Mader and Calhoun in 2000 proposed a more comprehensive classification for osteomyelitis [8]. This is also known as Cierny-Mader classification [8].

This was based upon the following [8]:

a) *The anatomy of the bone infection*: Based on the anatomic involvement of the bone.

b) *The physiology of the host* [8].

According to this classification, the disease was divided into four stages. These stages combined four anatomical disease types and three physiological host categories. This resulted in the description of 12 discrete clinical stages of osteomyelitis [8].

Classification and staging system of Osteomyelitis of the jaws developed by Cierny *et al.* and Vibhagool (1992) [16]

{Taken from Osteomyelitis of jaws by Baltenspenger and Eyrich-2009}

I. Anatomic Types

Stage 1: Medullary Osteomyelitis – It is confined to the medullary bone. There is no cortical involvement. It usually occurs due to hematogenous spread.

Stage 2: Superficial Osteomyelitis – It involves less than 2 cm bony defect. It only involves cortical bone. The defect does not involve cancellous bone. It usually occurs by direct inoculation of contiguous focus of infection.

Stage 3: Localised Osteomyelitis – It involves less than 2 cm bony defect radiographically without the involvement of both the cortices. The bone is stable.

Stage 4: Diffuse Osteomyelitis – It involves defect greater than 2 cm of the bone or entire thickness of the bone. There may be pathologic fracture and non-union with instability of the bone.

II. Physiologic Classification

A Host: normal host

B Host: host which is systemically (Bs) or locally (Bl) compromised

C Host: treatment worse than the disease. These are those patients which are so severely compromised that the radical treatment necessary is unacceptable on the basis of risk-benefit ratio.

III. Systemic/Local Factors that Affect Immune Surveillance, Metabolism, and Local Vascularity

a) *Systemic (Bs)*

Malnutrition, Renal or hepatic failure, Diabetes mellitus, Chronic hypoxia, Immune deficiency/suppression, Malignancy, Extremes of age, Autoimmune disease, Tobacco & alcohol abuse.

b) *Local (Bl)*

Chronic lymph edema, Venous stasis, Major vessel disease, Arteritis, Extensive scarring, Radiation fibrosis, Small vessel disease, Loss of local sensation.

Disadvantage: Although this classification system helps the clinician for the formulation of treatment strategies for each stage due to stratification of the infection as explained above, it is considered unnecessarily complex and impractical as well while dealing with infections of the maxillofacial region [8]. The oral cavity is unique since it beers teeth and connects the jaw bone to the teeth with the periodontium [8]. Hence, osteomyelitis of the jaws differs from osteomyelitis of long bones in several important aspects [8].

It is of interest to know that the etiopathogenesis of a disease can be determined by specific local immunological and microbiological aspects [8]. These further have an impact on the treatment of the disease too. Based on these facts, there is limited possibility to extrapolate the facts of classification of long bone infections to disease of the jaws [8]. In consideration to the fact that the osteomyelitis of the jaws is a clinical entity of long standing recognition, several authors have proposed different classification systems for the osteomyelitis of the maxillofacial region as well [8]. It is supported by the fact that it differs from the osteomyelitis of the long bones in many aspects.

Following is an overview of the most commonly cited classifications of maxillofacial osteomyelitis: (Table **1-4**).

Table 1. Classification systems described in the literature for osteomyelitis of the jaws [8].
[From Osteomyelitis of jaws by Baltenspenger and Eyrich in 2009]

Reference	Classification	Classification criteria

Hudson JW
 	
Osteomyelitis of the jaws: a 50-year perspective.
 	
J Oral Maxillofac Surg 1993 Dec;
 	
51(12):1294-301
	I. **ACUTE FORMS OF OSTEOMYELITIS**
	(Suppurative or Nonsuppurative)
	  A. Contagious focus
	    1. Trauma
	    2. Surgery
	    3. Odontogenic Infection
	  B. Progressive
	    1. Burns
	    2. Sinusitis
	    3. Vascular insufficiency
	  C. Hematogenous (metastatic)
	    1. Developing skeleton (children)
	  II. **CHRONIC FORMS OF OSTEOMYELITIS**
	  A. Recurrent multifocal
	    1. Developing skeleton (children)
	    2. Escalated osteogenic activity (< age 25 years)
	  B. Garre's
	    1. Unique proliferative Subperiosteal reaction
	    2. Developing skeleton (children and young adults)
	  C. Suppurative or nonsuppurative
	    1. Inadequately treated forms
	    2. Systemically compromised forms
	    3. Refractory forms (chronic recurrent multifocal osteomyelitis)
	  D. Diffuse sclerosing
	    1. Fastidious microorganisms
	    2. Compromised host/pathogen Interface
		Classification based on clinical picture and radiology.
		
		The two major groups (acute and chronic osteomyelitis) are differentiated by the clinical course of the disease after onset, relative to surgical and antimicrobial therapy. The arbitrary time limit of 1 month is used to differentiate acute from chronic osteomyelitis **(Marx 1991, Mercuri 1991, Koorbusch 1992).**

Table 2. Classification systems described in the literature for osteomyelitis of the jaws [8].

Reference	Classification	Classification criteria
Hudson JW Osteomyelitis of the jaws: a 50-year perspective. *J Oral Maxillofac Surg 1993 Dec;51(12):1294-301*	I. Hematogenous osteomyelitis II. Osteomyelitis secondary to a contiguous focus of infection III. Osteomyelitis associated with or without peripheral vascular disease	Classification based on pathogenesis. **From Vibhagool 1993**
Hudson JW Osteomyelitis of the jaws: a 50-year perspective. *J Oral Maxillofac Surg 1993 Dec;51(12):1294-301*	**I. Anatomic Types** **Stage I:** Medullary osteomyelitis – involved medullary bone without cortical involvement; usually hematogenous **Stage II:** Superficial osteomyelitis – less than 2 cm bony defect without cancellous bone **Stage III**: Localized osteomyelitis – less than 2 cm bony defect on radiograph, defect does not appear to involve both cortices **Stage IV:** Diffuse osteomyelitis – defect greater than 2 cm. Pathologic fracture, infection, nonunion **II. Physiological class** A : Normal host B : Systemic compromised host, Local compromised host C : Treatment worse than disease	Dual classification based on pathological anatomy and pathophysiology **From Vibhagool 1993 and Cierny 1985**
Mittermayer CH ***Schattauer, Stuttgart-New York 1976***	**I. Acute suppurative osteomyelitis** (rarefactional osteomyelitis) **II. Chronic suppurative osteomyelitis (sclerosing osteomyelitis)** **III. Chronic focal sclerosing osteomyelitis** (pseudo-paget, condensing osteomyelitis) **IV. Chronic diffuse sclerosing osteomyelitis** **V. Chronic osteomyelitis with proliferative periostitis** (Garrè's chronic non-suppurative sclerosing osteitis, ossifying periostitis) **VI. Specific osteomyelitis** 1. Tuberculous osteomyelitis 2. Syphilitic osteomyelitis 3. Actinomycotic osteomyelitis	Classification based on clinical picture, radiology, pathology, and etiology

Table 3. Classification systems described in the literature for osteomyelitis of the jaws [8].

Reference	Classification	Classification criteria
Hjorting-Hansen E Decortication in treatment of osteomyelitis of the mandible. *OOO 1970:May;29(5):641-55*	I. Acute/subacute osteomyelitis II. Secondary chronic osteomyelitis III. Primary chronic osteomyelitis	*Classification based on clinical picture and radiology*

Marx RE
Chronic Osteomyelitis of the Jaws
Oral &Maxillofacial Surgery Clinics of North America, Vol 3, No 2, May 91, 367-81
Mercuri LG
Acute Osteomyelitis of the Jaws
Oral & Maxillofacial Surgery Clinics of North America, Vol 3, No 2, May 91,
355-65
	I. Acute osteomyelitis
	  1. Associated with Hematogenous spread
	  2. Associated with intrinsic bone pathology or peripheral vascular disease
	  3. Associated with odontogenic & nonodontogenic local processes
	II. Chronic osteomyelitis
	1. Chronic recurrent multifocal Osteomyelitis of children
	2. Garrè's osteomyelitis
	3. Chronic suppurative osteomyelitis
	  – Foreign body related
	  – Systemic disease related
	  – Related to persistent or resistant organisms
	4. True chronic diffuse sclerosing Osteomyelitis
		Classification based on clinical picture, radiology, etiology, and pathophysiology
		Classification of acute osteomyelitis by **Mercuri**,
		Classification of chronic osteomyelitis by **Marx**.
		The arbitrary time limit of 1 month is used to differ acute from chronic osteomyelitis
		*From **Waldvogel and Medoff** 1970*

Panders AK, Hadders HN
 	
Chronic sclerosing inflammations of the jaw.
 	
Osteomyelitis sicca (Garre), Chronic sclerosing osteomyelitis with fine-meshed trabecular structure, and very dense sclerosing osteomyelitis.
 	
OOO 1970 Sep;30(3):396-412
	I. Primarily chronic jaw inflammation
	  1. Osteomyelitis sicca (synonymous osteomyelitis of Garrè, chronic sclerosing nonsuppurative osteomyelitis of Garrè, periostitis ossificans)
	  2. Chronic sclerosing osteomyelitis with fine-meshed trabecular structure
	  3. Local and more extensive ver dense sclerosing osteomyelitis
	II. Secondary chronic jaw inflammation
	III. Chronic specific jaw inflammations
	  – Tuberculosis
	  – Syphilis
	  – Lepra
	  – Actinomycosis
		Classification based on clinical picture and radiology
		
		Classification of chronic osteomyelitis forms only

Table 4. Classification systems described in the literature for osteomyelitis of the jaws [8]

Reference	Classification	Classification criteria
Schelhorn P, Zenk W [*Clinics and therapy of the osteomyelitis of the lower jaw*]. *Stomatol DDR 1989 Oct;39(10):672-6*	**I. Acute osteomyelitis** **II. Secondary chronic osteomyelitis** **III. Primary chronic osteomyelitis** **IV. Special forms** – Osteomyelitis sicca – Chronic sclerosing osteomyelitis Garrè	*Based on clinical picture*
Topazian RG *Osteomyelitis of the Jaws. In Topizan RG,* *Goldberg MH (eds): Oral and Maxillofacial* *Infections.* *Philadelphia, WB Saunders 1994,* *Chapter 7, pp 251-88*	**I. Suppurative osteomyelitis** 1. Acute suppurative osteomyelitis 2. Chronic suppurative osteomyelitis – Primary chronic suppurative osteomyelitis – Secondary chronic suppurative osteomyelitis 3. Infantile osteomyelitis **II. Nonsuppurative osteomyelitis** 1. Chronic sclerosing osteomyelitis – Focal sclerosing osteomyelitis – Diffuse sclerosing osteomyelitis 2. Garrè's sclerosing osteomyelitis 3. Actinomycotic osteomyelitis 4. Radiation osteomyelitis and necrosis	*Based on clinical picture, radiology, and etiology* *(specific forms such as syphilitic, tuberculous, brucellar, viral, chemical, Escherichia coli and Salmonella osteomyelitis not integrated in classification)*
Bernier S, Clermont S, Maranda G, **Turcotte JY** *Osteomyelitis of the jaws.* *J Can Dent Assoc 1995 May;61(5):441-2,* *445-8*	**I. Suppurative osteomyelitis** 1. Acute suppurative osteomyelitis 2. Chronic suppurative osteomyelitis **II. Nonsuppurative osteomyelitis** 1. Chronic focal sclerosing osteomyelitis 2. Chronic diffuse sclerosing osteomyelitis 3. Garrè's chronic sclerosing osteomyelitis(proliferative osteomyelitis) **III. Osteoradionecrosis**	*Based on clinical and Radiological picture*
Wassmund M **Lehrbuch der praktischen Chirurgie des Mundes und der Kiefer.** *Meusser, Leipzig 1935*	**I. Exudative osteitis** **II. Resorptive osteitis** **III. Productive osteitis** **IV. Acute necrotizing osteitis** (osteomyelitis) **V. Chronic osteomyelitis** 1. Chronic course of an acute osteomyelitis 2. Occult osteomyelitis 3. Chronic necrotizing osteomyelitis with hypertrophy 4. Chronic exudative osteomyelitis 5. Productive osteomyelitis	*Based on clinical picture and radiology* *(note that classification was developed before introduction of antibiotic therapy)*

It is of interest to know that however there are a lot of classification systems of osteomyelitis of the jaws as described above in the literature, the clinician or the dental professional still come across difficulty in classifying this disease particularly of mandible.

According to **Suei** *et al.* **in 2005** there are two basic difficulties faced by the dental professional while diagnosing and classifying a case especially of mandibular osteomyelitis [22]. One difficulty is that classification systems are found to be inconsistent and moreover they differ among the references [22, 23]. Due to this fact, the clinicians and researchers are not able to develop a better and more comprehensive understanding of this particular disease [21].

These facts have led to a dilemma amongst the professionals to decide whether the classification which they follow is appropriate for their treatment planning strategies. Further a similar dilemma also exists among the academicians while training students and designing clinical research in this context [22]. **Kahn** *et al.* **in 1994, Suei** *et al.* **in 1996 and 2005** observed that the second difficulty observed is regarding SAPHO (Synovitis, acne, pustulosis, hypertosis, and osteitis) syndrome [22]. According to them the existing classification systems of the osteomyelitis of jaws failed in identifying SAPHO syndrome as a distinct entity [22, 24].

According to **Suei** *et al.* **in 2005**, proposed Classification for Mandibular Osteomyelitis was divided into two distinct conditions [22].

a. Bacterial osteomyelitis and

b. Osteomyelitis in SAPHO syndrome

This classification was based on the etiology, presence/absence of pus, radiological findings, histological characteristics and response of the patient to antibiotic therapy. Further the authors also considered the prognosis and complications of the disease as well [22] (Table **5**).

Table 5. Proposed classification and clinicopathologic findings of mandibular osteomyelitis [22].

	Bacterial Osteomyelitis	Osteomyelitis in SAPHO syndrome
Synonyms	(Acute) suppurative (Chronic) suppurative Secondary chronic	(Chronic) diffuse sclerosing, Chronic sclerosing, Primary chronic, Osteomyelitis sicca, Chronic sclerosing nonsuppurative, chronic recurrent multifocal
Cause	Bacterial infection	Unknown

(Table 5) cont.....

	Bacterial Osteomyelitis	**Osteomyelitis in SAPHO syndrome**
Sex	Male predominance	Female predominance
Pain/Swelling	Yes	Yes
Suppuration	Yes	No
Radiographic Findings	Osteolytic pattern Sequestrum formation.	Mixed pattern, Solid type pattern External bone resorption, bone enlargement
Histologic Findings	Inflammation of bone, abscess, necrotic tissue, sequester formation	Inflammation of bone, reactive hyperplasia of bone, resemblance to fibrous dysplasia
Antibiotic therapy	Effective	Not effective (anti-inflammatory drugs including corticosteroids and pamidronate t/t are recommended)
Prognosis	Good (cured within six months)	Poor (often continues for more than six months)
Complications	None	Osteomyelitis/arthritis at the other bone/joints, skin diseases (palmoplantar pustulosis, pustular psoriasis, acne)

1. **Bacterial Osteomyelitis**: Cause is Bacteria. Clinically presents with Pain, Swelling and Suppuration which are characteristic to Bacterial infection [22].
2. **Osteomyelitis in SAPHO Syndrome:** It represents a systemic disease which is characterized by a number of clinical features which includes combination of osteomyelitis, arthritis, and skin diseases (pustulosis, psoriasis, and acne) [22].

The Zurich Classification System [8]

This system of classification was developed at the **Department of Cranio-Maxillofacial Surgery of University of Zurich**. It is a hierarchical classification system which is based on clinical appearance, course of disease and radiological features [8].

According to this classification, there are three major groups of Osteomyelitis of jaws [8].

1. Acute Osteomyelitis (AO)
2. Secondary Chronic Osteomyelitis (SCO)
3. Primary Chronic Osteomyelitis (PCO)

According to **Eyrich and Baltensperger in 2003**, Primary chronic osteomyelitis is chronic non-suppurative osteomyelitis. When it occurs in children and adolescents it is termed as Garre's osteomyelitis [8, 22]. The histopathological picture is considered as secondary classification criterion, taking into account that findings are mostly unspecific and non-conclusive. According to them, histopathology is considered as a gold standard in case of dilemma [8].

A tertiary criterion is the further sub-classification of these major osteomyelitis groups which is based on etiology and pathogenesis of disease. Interestingly these tertiary criteria are quite helpful in determining the necessary therapeutic strategies. These therapeutic strategies may differ among the subgroups [8].

An overview of the Zurich classification of osteomyelitis of the jaws and the classification criteria [8] are given in Fig. (**4.1** and Table **6**).

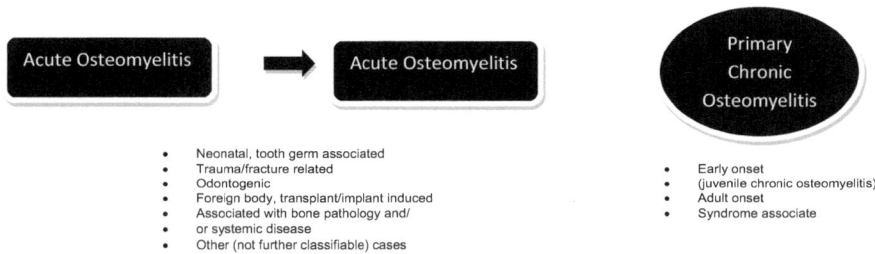

Fig. (4.1). The Zurich classification of osteomyelitis of the jaws [8]. (*From Osteomyelitis of jaws by Baltensperger MM and Eyrich GK-2009*).

Table 6. Criteria of Zurich classification of osteomyelitis [8]

Hierarchic order of classification criteria	Classification criteria	Classificaton
First	Clinical appearance and course of disease Radiology	**Major groups** Acute osteomyelitis (AO) Secondary chronic osteomyelitis (SCO) Primary chronic osteomyelitis (PCO)
Second	Pathology (gross pathology and histology)	Differentiation of cases that cannot clearly be distinguished solely on clinical appearance and course of the disease; important for exclusion of differential diagnosis in borderline cases.
Third	Etiology Pathogenesis	Subgroups of AO, SCO, and PCO

CHAPTER 5

Imaging Modalities

Abstract: Osteomyelitis is an inflammatory disease of bone. It occurs because of infection by pathogenic microorganisms. According to various authors, the disease may present as alveolar osteitis if only the alveolar bone is involved. On the contrary it is considered as osteomyelitis when the infection reaches the marrow cavity of the bone. However the disease presents various clinical features, it is sometimes difficult to diagnose this disease on the basis of clinical presentation alone. Further, delay in the diagnosis leads to progression of the disease. This can be avoided with the help of radiographic evaluation. Radiographically, the location or anatomical involvement of the affected site may help to differentiate between alveolar osteitis and osteomyelitis. Histolopathologically localized alveolar osteitis may present the same features as alveolar osteomyelitis. This may be attributed to the fact that alveolar bone possesses bone marrow too. Researchers also stressed on the early diagnosis and adequate treatment for osteomyelitis failing which, acute osteomyelitis may progress to subacute or chronic stage. Henceforth imaging modalities play a crucial role in the early diagnosis of the osteomyelitis of jaws. Various radiographic and imaging modalities which can prove to be beneficial in osteomyelitis of jaws are conventional radiography, CT Scan (Computed Tomography), MRI (Magnetic Resonance Imaging) and Ultrasonography to name a few. Researchers even quote that Nuclear medicine imaging is able to detect osteomyelitic changes 10 to 14 days in advance to their appearance on plain radiographs.

Keywords: Alveolar osteitis, Conventional Radiographs, CT Scan, Early diagnosis, Imaging Modalities, MRI, Nuclear Medicine imaging, Orthopentomography, Osteomyelitis, Ultrasonography.

ROLE OF IMAGING

It is a well known fact that imaging modalities play a vital role in the early diagnosis as well as follow up of inflammatory conditions of the bone and maxillofacial region. Different type of radiographic techniques and other imaging modalities are used by different authors in the literature [25 - 28].

Worth & Stoneman in 1977 stated that conventional radiology is good for Osteomyelitis diagnosis which can be supplemented by computed tomography when required [28]. **Yoshiura *et al*. in 1994** recommended that CT scan can help to determine the extent of the lesion [27]. Certain authors like **Aliabadi *et al*.** in

1994 [28] also recommended the use of MRI and radionuclide bone scanning in addition to conventional radiography and CT for early diagnosis of the disease [24 - 28]. **Topazian** believed that proper imaging helps to determine the extent and degree of the disease [1]. It may also help to precisely locate the position of the sequestra and thereby planning the approach and extent of the surgery [8]. Imaging also helps to determine when treatment may be stopped [1].

According to **Yoshiura *et al.* in 1994** and **Taori *et al.* in 2005**, the following is the significance of radiological evaluation in osteomyelitis.

a) To differentiate osteomyelitis from the diseases having similar clinical signs and symptoms [28] and

b) To evaluate the progress of the disease and its response to the treatment [1].

Imaging helps the clinician to achieve the following goals [8]:

1. Confirmation of the presence of infection or inflammation in the upper or lower jaw/maxillofacial region [8].
2. Recognition of a predisposing bony condition or a local infection source [1, 8, 26].
3. To delineate the anatomical location as well as the extent of the bony involvement. It also helps to define the involvement of potential associated soft tissues [29].
4. Differentiate osteomyelitis from the other lesions with similar clinical features [27 - 29].
5. To identify whether the maxillofacial lesions are due to any associated syndrome or any multifocal inflammatory process [8].
6. Recognize the complications which may arise during the natural course of the disease or during the treatment plan.

IMAGING TECHNIQUES

A. Conventional Radiography

This is a technique for initial screening. According to **Coviello and Stevens in 2007**, there is a late change in plain/conventional radiographs for early disease confined to the marrow spaces [30]. The simplest intraoral radiographic technique used for initial screening followed by most of the clinicians is an intra oral periapical radiograph (IOPA) which may be supplemented by an occlusal radiograph. The limitation is the limited anatomical region covered. Among the extra oral conventional radiographs, the panoramic view is of prime importance. It helps to evaluate the dentition, status of osseous confines and internal structures of the jaw [8]. It also serves as an adequate basis for the follow-up examination of such patients (Fig. **5.1**). The panoramic view can also be supplemented by intraoral radiographs [8].

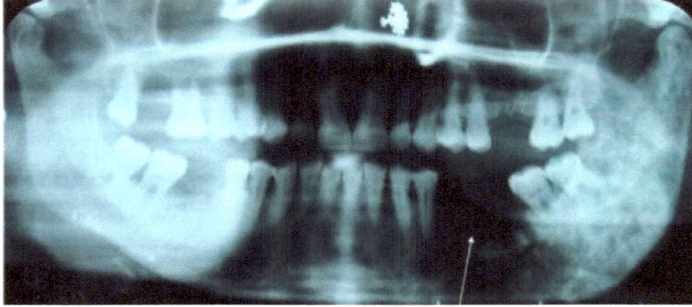

Fig. (5.1). Conventional Orthopantomogram highlighting distended left mandibular body and ramus with the involvement of mandibular condyle. Internal structure reveals mixed radiolucent and radiopaque lesion on the left side with the presence of bony sequestra.

Even though the conventional panoramic radiographs are still prescribed by dental professionals, **Kashima *et al.* in 1990** reviewed and studied their role in digital format as well (Fig. **5.2**).

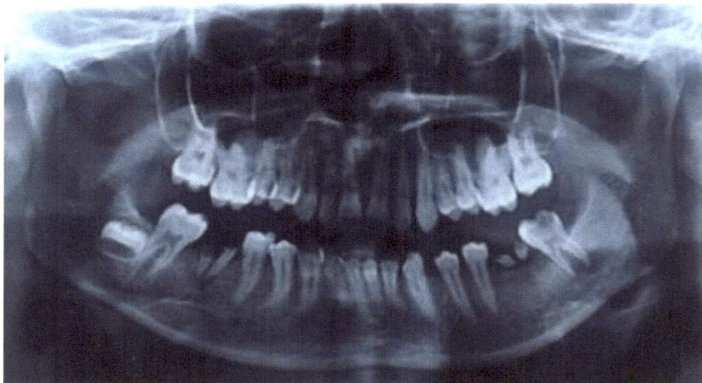

Fig. (5.2). Digital OPG of a patient revealing radiolucency at the periapical region of 37 due to pulpal involvement.

These digital panoramic radiographs are of high diagnostic value and produce less blurring [31]. **Schuknecht B in 2009** [8] stated that the panoramic radiograph exposes the patient with less radiation dose of 0.3 mSv [8]. Sometimes additional conventional radiographs are also recommended to focus specific anatomical areas of the maxillofacial region. These are: The mandibular lateral oblique view provides a better unilateral projection of mandibular body [8]. The occlusal view

(Fig. **5.3**) helps to provide a depiction of the symphysis and maxilla area. Clementschitsch stated that the posteroanterior view (PA view) of the mandible is of great value to delineate the mandibular condyle [8]. Waters view is deemed best for the depiction of the maxillary sinuses [8].

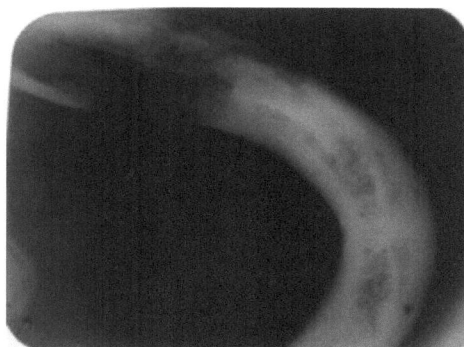

Fig. (5.3). Mandibular Lateral Occlusal view revealing radiolucency in the body of left side extending from buccal to lingual cortical plate.

Worth and Stoneman in 1977 stated that conventional radiographs may fail to reveal any radiographic changes for the initial 4−8 days. **Aliabadi and Nikpoor in 1994** stated that the disease becomes evident on the radiographs after 14 days of onset [26].

According to **Worth and Stoneman in 1977,** an estimated 30% - 50% of the mineralized portion of the bone must be destroyed before significant radiographic changes can be distinguished [1]. This degree of bone alteration requires a minimum of 4 days and up to 14 days after the onset of acute osteomyelitis. **Davis and Carr in 1990** advocated that the full extent of bone dissolution cannot be determined radiographically until 3 weeks after the onset of the symptoms. Radiographic changes clearly lag behind the actual clinical situation in the early as well as in the late stages of the disease process [1].

Once osteomyelitis has become well established, radiographic changes usually demonstrate one of the following groups of characteristics described by Worth [1]

1. Scattered areas of bone destruction that vary in size and number which are separated by variable distances and by bone with normal or nearly normal appearance. Bone has a moth eaten appearance [8]. This may be attributed to enlargement of medullary spaces and widening of the Volkmann's canals resulting from bony destruction by lysis and replacement with granulation tissue.

2. Bone destruction with varying extent in which there are bony sequestra (Fig. **5.4**) with evidence of a trabecular pattern and marrow spaces. A sheath of a new bone often is found, separated from sequestra by a zone of radiolucency [1].

3. Stippled or granular densification of bone caused by subperiosteal deposition of new bone on surfaces of existing trabecuale at the expense of marrow spaces. The central sequestra usually present in osteomyelitis help to distinguish it from fibrous dysplasia.

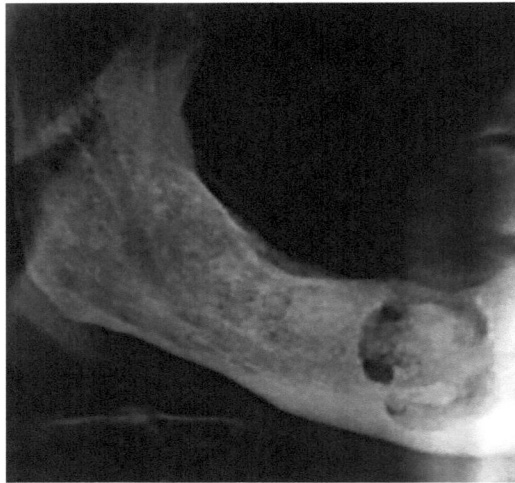

Fig. (5.4). Cropped OPG of a patient revealing "sequestrum" bordered by a radiolucent zone.

Schuknecht *et al.* in 1997 compared conventional radiographs and CT regarding osteomyelitis. According to them, plain films were interpreted normal in 75% of the patients within the first 2 weeks. Only 37.5% showed pathological changes on the radiographs within 4 weeks of initiation of symptoms. On the contrary, the radiographs will definitely show pathological changes within and after the fourth week [8].

The clinician or a student can diagnose Osteomyelitis on the radiographs on the basis of following [8]:

a. Loss of bony trabeculae in relation to the empty socket of the extracted tooth. This may present as the initial sign of the disease. This may present grossly as a focal area of radiolucency [8].

b. Widening of periodontal ligament space or a defect/loss of the lamina dura [8].

c. Destruction of bone. The destruction of bone starts with the involvement of cancellous bone. Progressive resorption of bone may lead to involvement of cortical plates due to increase in pressure exerted by the inflammatory process.

d. Erosion of the endosteal margin of the basal mandibular cortical bone or effacement of the contour of the alveolar maxillary recess may prove as the additional early signs of the disease [8].

On the basis of the above said features, it can be rightly said that conventional radiographs are sometimes able to delineate potential Odontogenic source of infection even though they are frequently negative to access the initial stages of the disease [8] (Fig. **5.1-5.4**).

On the contrary, conventional radiographs can serve as a good radiological tool to access the patient during advanced stages. During advanced stages, the patient may present with Sequestra (Fig. **5.4, 5.5**) and/or periosteal bone formation which can serve as radiological "indicator" and can thus play a significant role to arrive at the diagnosis [8]. A periosteal reaction is rare in the maxilla while it may affect all the non-alveolar borders of the mandible [8, 26]. It is well evident on conventional radiographs. It can present as single layered linear radiopaque line separated by radiolucent line from the cortical bone of the mandible. Such periosteal bone formation is more pronounced in younger age group. It can be attributed to the fact that the there is more osteogenic potential in younger patients. Further it is comparatively easier for the periosteum to get stripped off from the mandibular cortex in younger age [8].

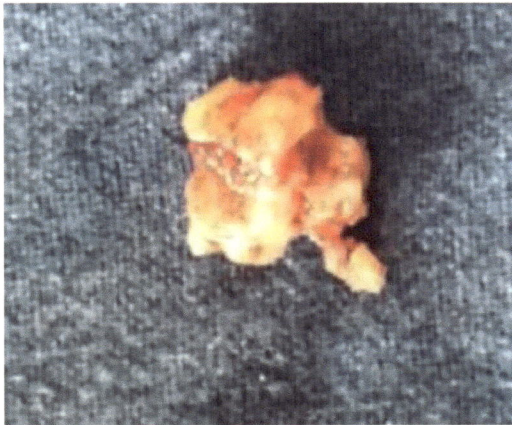

Fig. (5.5). Sequestra removed from the patient.

Several authors like **Aliabadi and Nikpoor in 1994**, were also of the same view that elevation of periosteum and areas of poorly defined radiolucency are the earliest radiographic changes of the bone in children [26]. Elevation of periosteum can further result in periosteal bone reaction which is particularly more prominent in children as dictated earlier in this chapter [26]. The elevated periosteum lays down bone to form the "involucrum" [8]. The involucrum can partially or completely surround the bone [26]. Periosteal new bone formation can best be visualized on the Lateral oblique or panoramic radiographs when it occurs along the inferior aspect of the mandible [1, 8].

Furthermore, according to **Ida *et al.* in 1997** and **Schuknecht *et al.* in 1997**, CT scan shows a higher incidence of periosteal reactions as compared to conventional films. This holds true for osseous fistulae as well. Henceforth in favour of early application of CT or MRI examination, most of the plain films except panoramic radiographs are not in use in context of diagnosing periosteal bone reaction [8].

B. Computed Tomography and Magnetic Resonance Imaging

CT and MRI are considered as advanced imaging modalities to capture detailed anatomical extension of the disease. Since these modalities provide high-resolution morphological information of the bony and soft tissue structures, they have attained significant importance over the past 2 decades [8, 32 - 36]. Since these are cross sectional imaging techniques, they are able to avoid over projection of structures in the second dimension. Hence they differ from conventional radiographs, which are referred to as "projectional techniques" [8].

COMPUTED TOMOGRAPHY

Examination Technique

It utilizes a fan shaped beam of collimated radiation. It is applied with continuous motion during which scanning region is also moved. The resultant images are reconstructed from a spiral CT data set [8]. These images allow the clinician to assess the maxillofacial region in oro-vestibular (antero-posterior), baso-alveolar (supero-inferior) and mesio-distal dimension [8] by reconstruction of axial, coronal and sagittal planes that too usually from one data set acquired in the axial plane. **Coviello and Stevens in 2005** advocated the role of CT in osteomyelitis of jaws [30]. CT is well suited and is considered gold standard to highlight periosteal bone reactions due to its higher sensitivity in detecting early changes of bone in cases of acute osteomyelitis [8].

A spiral, cranio-caudal acquisition with thin collimation (0.5–1.0 mm) is obtained covering the maxilla and the mandible to the hyoid bone with the patient in a supine position. For reconstructions in the axial and coronal plane, the beam is angulated parallel to mandibular body and along the mandibular ramus respectively [8].

Since CT is well known to delineate bony structures, a contrast medium is required in case the soft tissue details are required along with. Henceforth when facial and masticator spaces are analysed for infection/inflammation, intravenous application of iodine-containing contrast material is carried out which is performed with 100 ml at a flow rate of 2 ml/s [8].

Findings

According to **Osborn *et al.* in 1982**, Computed Tomography can be very well used to evaluate the presence of osteomyelitis [8].

Merkesteyn *et al.* in 1988 stated that CT is used to evaluate the presence as well as extent of mandibular osteomyelitis (Fig. **5.6**).

Further **Ida *et al.* in 2005** advocated the role of CT in the evaluation of accompanying soft tissue inflammation in addition to the previous indications. However, the role of CT in patients suspected of harbouring osteomyelitis of the mandible was advocated by **van Merkesteyn *et al.* in 1988** after latency.

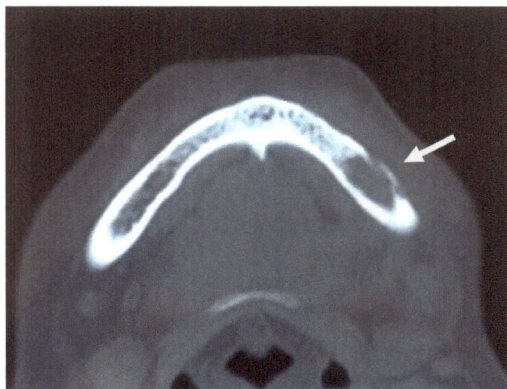

Fig. (5.6). Axial CT scan section of the molar region showing destruction of the buccal cortical bone.

Ida *et al.* in 2005 and various other authors stated that CT helps in early detection of osteomyelitis due to soft tissue information [8].

CT scan may present the following features regarding osteomyelitis of jaws [26] (According to **Aliabadi and Nikpoor in 1994**):

1. Medullary portion of the involved bone reveals increased attenuation value even if there is no radiographic changes.
2. There can be destruction of cortical bone (Fig. **5.6**) [37] or evidence of new bone formation.
3. Constriction of the medullary cavity.

4. Demonstration of sequestra and/or evidence of intraosseous gas [26].

The presence of intraosseous gas on CT scan was also documented by another researcher named **Ram *et al.* in 1981** as a sign of osteomyelitis. Some of the authors like **Pineda *et al.* in 2009**, has even graded CT scans superior to MRI for detection of sequestra, cloacas, involucra, or intraosseous gas.

CT scan also aids to perform needle biopsies and joint aspiration [38, 39]. On the other hand, according to **Coviello and Stevens in 2007**, the overall soft tissue contrast resolution of CT is inferior to that of MRI for delineation of abscess cavities or fistulae [38, 39]. **Cierny *et al.* in 2003** mentioned the disadvantage of metallic objects in the area of interest like screws and restorations during CT examination. **Bohndorf in 2004** mentioned that there can be significant loss of image resolution due to the presence of metals like amalgam restorations, clasps *etc* in or near the area of osteomyelitis. This can be attributed to beam hardening artefact [38 - 42].

MAGNETIC RESONANCE IMAGING

Aliabadi and Nikpoor in 1994 stressed that MRI can be recognized as a useful modality [43] in evaluation of maxillofacial osteomyelitis. It is due to the ability of MRI machine to image the anatomical structure in multiple planes with excellent soft tissue contrast [26]. Several authors like **Tang *et al.* in 1988** and **Gold *et al.* in 1991** [26 - 32] have highlighted that the specificity as well as sensitivity of MRI for detecting Osteomyelitis was in the range of 89-100 %.

Examination Technique

The technique of Magnetic resonance imaging is not based upon radiation exposure [8]. On the contrary, it is based on proton relaxation within a static high magnetic field. T1 relaxation is based on longitudinal relaxation while T2 effects are based on transverse relaxation. It is the T1 image which will provide the basis for assessment of contrast enhancement and displays fluid as hypointense (dark) signal. It further consists of a coronal and axial fast T2-weighted series that covers the upper and lower jaw with a slice thickness of 3.5 mm. T2 effects are indicated by increased hyperintense (bright) signal within fluid and oedema and are not combined with contrast agent [8].

The contrast agent used in MRI is gadolinium (Gd) [8]. Gadolinium has the tendency to shorten the T1 relaxation time. Consequently, when the blood tissue barrier is disturbed, it will lead to a high signal (bright) within tissue [8]. This enhancement by the usage of contrast agent occurs in the case of infection, inflammation or trauma [1]. It may also happen in the cases of tumors and also helps to delineate the extent and exact location of involvement [8].

Aliabadi and Nikpoor in 1994 stated that MRI is very sensitive in diagnosing early medullary changes of the bone [8, 26]. Henceforth it may help to diagnose osteomyelitis at a very early stage as compared to conventional radiographs and CT scan.

This high sensitivity of MRI is attributed to the availability of mobile protons within medullary fat for any process that affects the cancellous bone after extending over the confines of cortical bone [8]. Inflammation of the marrow leads to increase in water content. This results in abundant mobile protons which further leads to bright signal on T2 images and low signal on T1. It also leads to contrast enhancement. Henceforth, the sensitivity of MRI surpasses CT in regards to cancellous bone extension, as well as recognition of non-calcified periosteal reactions [8].

Findings

Tang *et al.* **in 1988** and **Aliabadi in 1994** recommended the use of MRI to evaluate suspected cases of Osteomyelitis [42]. It was attributed to its ability to demonstrate [42] changes in the water content of bone marrow that too with an excellent structural definition and spatial resolution [38, 44]. **Kocher in 2006** revealed that MRI is even sensitive to detect osteomyelitis within 3 to 5 days of onset of infection [38, 45].

According to **Jevtic in 2004**, the advantages of MRI go far beyond the diagnosis. It helps the operating surgeon regarding the optimal surgical treatment planning [38]. It also helps to evaluate the extent of devitalized tissue involved that would require modified management to avoid morbidity and complications.

According to **Pineda** *et al.* **in 2009**, initial MRI screening usually includes T1-weighted and T2-weighted spin-echo pulse sequences. Different pulse sequences and imaging protocols can be used in the evaluation of the musculoskeletal system [38]. Depending on the pulse sequences used, major differences can be noted on the signal intensity and appearance of normal and abnormal tissues (Fig. **5.7**).

According to **Aliabadi and Nikpoor in 1994**, the combination of short-tau inversion- recovery (STIR) and T1 spin echo sequences results in high sensitivity and specificity of MRI for the detection of osteomyelitis [38]. This obviates the need for any additional radiological examination for diagnostic purpose [26, 38].

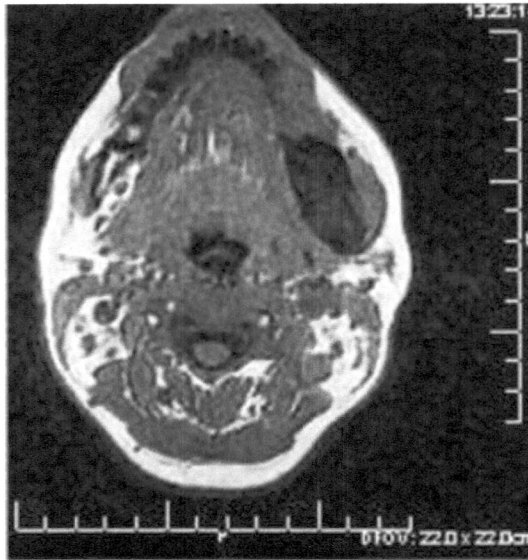

Fig. (5.7). MRI revealing expansion of the left side of the body and ramus of mandible with altered signal intensity which was hypotensive with replacement of bone marrow.

MRI findings in osteomyelitis on different type of sequences are as follows [38]:

a. The edema and exudates within the medullary space produce an ill-defined low-signal intensity on the T1-weighted images. On the contrary they will produce a high signal on T2-weighted as well as on STIR or fat- suppressed sequences [38, 46].

b. A sequestrum is visible as a low signal intensity structure on T1-weighted and STIR sequences. However the surrounding granulation tissue is intermediate to low signal intensity on T1-weighted images and high signal intensity with STIR or T2-weighted sequences [38].

c. With use of Gadolinium (intravenous contrast agent), the granulation tissue reveals enhancement while on the contrary, the sequestrum remains with low signal intensity.

d. The ossified periosteal shell and the dead tubular cortical bone of an involucrum have low signal intensity on all pulse sequences.

e. Periosteal reaction and cortical bone are separated by linear intermediate to high signal intensity on T2- weighted or STIR images [38].

f. A cloaca is perceived as a linear low signal intensity from periosteum that is elevated from the cortical bone or the thickened cortex that is interrupted by a high signal intensity gap on T2-weighted images [41]. According to **Santiago-Restrepo in 2003**, this high signal intensity can be seen extending into the soft tissues from the cloaca and may form a sinus tract or abscess.

g. Demonstration of increased signal intensity of the bone marrow on T2-weighted images may represent postsurgical or postinfectious granulation tissue and not necessarily persistent infection. However, serial magnetic resonance studies showing progression of this process in the marrow indicates the presence of active osteomyelitis.

Disadvantages of MRI are its occasional inability to distinguish infectious from reactive inflammation and difficulty in imaging sites with metallic implants, such as joint prostheses or fixation devices.

According to **Yamada** *et al.* **in 1995**, there is sequential involvement of the marrow in the angle and ramus up to the mandibular condyle. Due to osteomyelitis, there is increased replacement of hematopoietic tissue of marrow by fatty tissue [8]. This theoretically leads to the diagnosis of acute osteomyelitis easier in adolescents and adults compared with young children. In this age group more specific signs which leads to the diagnosis of osteomyelitis includes focal bone destruction, periosteal reaction and sequestra formation [8]. Some of the authors have also highlighted that MRI is less sensitive than CT in recognizing participation of compact bone in the early acute stages as compared to cancellous bone.

C. Cone Beam Computed Tomography

Cone Beam Computed Tomography (CBCT) is a new technique designed for dental and maxillofacial examinations. The technology, even though frequently also called as CT, is fundamentally quite different from CT. In CBCT, a cone-shaped radiation beam is rotated once around the region of interest in contrast to a fan shaped beam used in CT scan [8].

Limitations of the cone-beam technology consist of the inability to depict soft tissue, long data acquisition time from 18–36 s up to 75 s, and the low contrast resolution within compact bone.

According to Terzic, lower tube dosage is applied in CBCT. This significantly reduces the radiation dose to the patient. Effective radiation dose in CBCT is about 0.3 mSv. Since Cone Beam Computed Tomography is used to access hard tissue structures of the maxillofacial region, it has therefore gained considerable importance in the field of implantology, impacted third molars and the assessment of cysts. The ability of CBCT to detect osteomyelitis based on the evidence of irregular radiolucencies and osteosclerotic changes has recently been described by **Schulze** *et al.* **in 2006**. With the upcoming popularity and the rapid advances in cone-beam technology this imaging modality might show growing interest in the future [8].

D. Nuclear Medicine Imaging

It is a medical specialty rather than imaging modality. It involves the usage and application of certain radioactive substances for the diagnosis of a disease [8]. It is entirely different as compared to other imaging modalities. It can be attributed to the fact that it is considered as "endoradiology". This is so because it records the radiation which is being emitted from inside the body. This is in contrast to other radiographic modalities which are performed by exposure to X-rays generated by external sources. In addition, nuclear medicine scans are different from radiology as it is based on the function inspite of anatomy of the region scanned. Henceforth, it is referred to as a physiological imaging modality. Single Photon Emission Computed Tomography (SPECT) and Positron Emission Tomography (PET) scans are the two most common imaging modalities in nuclear medicine.

It is also known for its early diagnosis. As for as osteomyelitis is concerned, it can detect the changes 10 to 14 days before they are visible on plain radiographs [38]. It requires certain agents/radiopharmaceuticals to be administered either orally or injected intravenously to the patient. The agents that have been studied includes technetium-99m–labelled methylene diphosphonate (99mTc-MDP), gallium-67 citrate, and indium-111–labeled white blood cells *etc*. These agents are absorbed by the cells of the body which then emit radiation. This emitted radiation is then detected by external detectors (gamma cameras) which capture and form images. According to **Littenberg in 1992**, these agents are highly sensitive but have the inconvenience of low specificity to the disease [47]. Henceforth, it is difficult to differentiate osteomyelitis from certain other diseases and/or conditions such as fractures, neoplasia, or cellulitis [38]. Nuclear medicine scans may be a useful adjunctive study when x-rays are altered by pathologic or postsurgical changes.

a) Scintigraphy (Three Phase Bone Scintigraphy)

Scintigraphy utilizes internal radionuclides to create two-dimensional images. According to **Rohlin in 1993**, increased bone turnover activity is a sign of osteomyelitis in the initial stages. **Kohnlein *et al.* in 1997** stated that markedly increased bone turnover activity is indicated as an early sign in acute osteomyelitis [8].

According to **Reinert *et al.* in 1995**, increased bone turnover activity due to hyperaemia is detected as early as 2–3 days after the onset of symptoms [8]. According to **Rohlin in 1993**, the degree of uptake was reported as higher when plain films showed permeative bone destruction and areas of osteolysis compared with the moth-eaten or sclerotic appearance that prevails in chronic osteomyelitis.

According to **Kohnlein** *et al.* **in 1997**, with histology as reference to scintigraphy, the sensitivity in the acute phase is postulated to be close to 100% and false-negative results are attributed to the fact that the examination has been performed too early [8]. **Tsuchimochi** *et al.* **in 1991** reported that the drawbacks of scintigraphy in acute osteomyelitis are related to fact that distinction between soft tissue inflammation and bone involvement is limited. As a preoperative examination scintigraphy is not sufficient to determine the extent of mandibular osteomyelitis.

Heggie in 2000 postulated that it has to be complemented by an additional CT examination to provide the detailed osseous information required.

Scintigraphy: Basic Considerations

In the case of skeletal scintigraphy or bone scan, a radioactive tracer is injected into the circulation system. Most commonly 99mTc-labeled methylene diphosphonate is used a tracer and is administered intravenously.

According to **Pineda** *et al.* **in 2009**, the complete 99mTc bone scan consists of the following three phases:

i) Angiogram: It is the first phase and is also known as Flow study. In this, dynamic study of the region of interest is performed during the 60 seconds of injecting the tracer into the circulation.

ii) Blood Pool: This is the second phase and consists of static images performed a few minutes after injection. It will represent intravascular and extra vascular activity in the individual. This will aid for better spatial resolution between bone, joint and soft tissues.

iii) Bone Structures: This is the third phase and is performed 2 to 4 hours after injection of the tracer. It allows the demonstration the bony structures with good resolution.

Pineda *et al.* **in 2009** stated that when osteomyelitis is suspected, a three-phase bone scan should be performed. Further, the advantage of nuclear medicine is that it can even image patients with prostheses that too without an artefact. Since the injected tracer gets embed into the newly formed bone tissue, hence the uptake of the tracer is considered directly proportional to the osteoblastic activity of the bone. After administration of the tracer, the radiologist examines several consecutive phases of the scan. Acute osteomyelitis can be differentiated from chronic forms by a positive early phase in the former compared with negative early phases in the latter.

In an early phase (blood-pool study) soft tissue surrounding the infected bone can be assessed. This can give additional valuable information concerning involvement of these tissues in the infectious process.

Since the bone volume of the skeletal regions of the body in a healthy individual is different (According to **Hardt and Hofer in 1988**), henceforth the uptake of the radionuclide is higher in bone with larger mass than in delicate bony structures. As for as the maxillofacial region is concerned, the uptake is slightly higher in the maxilla and mandible compared with the rest of the skull. The predominant physiological factors are local tissue perfusion and regional metabolic activity. In the growing skeleton, the epiphyseal plates typically show increased activity.

The following criteria must always be addressed when interpreting a bone scan [8]:

a. Look for symmetrical uptake within the corresponding skeletal regions.
b. Regions with increased or decreased uptake compared with surrounding and corresponding bones are suspicious and may need further radiological investigation.
c. Increased uptake is a sign of increased metabolic activity. A physiological or decreased uptake indicates a normal osteoblastic bone activity or may be the result of a very aggressive lesion with failure of local bone repair.

As stated by **Hardt and Hofer in 1988**, the pathological bone conditions can lead to alterations in local blood flow and induce bone metabolism causing either increased resorption (osteolysis) or osteoblastic activity.

As long as the vascular supply to the centre and peripheral aspects of the bone lesion is maintained, an increased uptake is noted on the bone scan. However, if loss of bone is not repaired adequately, or local blood supply is compromised, the scintigraphic image will show a decreased uptake. An increased pathological uptake of radioactive tracer is noted in lesions which produce bone tissue, such as certain tumors. On the other hand, the uptake is increased by the processes which induce reparative bone reactions in the periphery of the lesion similar to cases of osteolytic metastasis. A decreased uptake is noted in lesions which eventually replace bony matrix without any or little repair. This can be observed in slow-growing pathologies such as cysts or odontogenic tumors.

b) Fluorine-18 Fluorodeoxyglucose Positron Emission Tomography

According to **Pineda *et al.* in 2009**, 18 -FDG is transported into cells *via* glucose transporters. Activated inflammatory cells demonstrate increased expression of glucose transporters.

As stated by **Stumpe and Strobel in 2006**, this technique has several potential advantages.

These are:

i. Results are available within 30- 60 minutes of tracer administration
ii. Imaging is not affected by metallic implant artefacts.
iii. It has a distinctly higher spatial resolution than do images obtained with single photon emitting tracers.
iv. It is less expensive than other nuclear medicine techniques.

It has been demonstrated by **Santiago-Restrepo in 2003** that FDG-PET has the highest diagnostic accuracy for confirming or excluding the diagnosis of chronic osteomyelitis in comparison to bone scintigraphy, MRI, or leukocyte scintigraphy.

Further, according to **Pineda in 2009**, the discussion of the application of PET in osteomyelitis is quite lively, but exceptionally scarce information is available for the use of 18FDG-PET in cases of osteomyelitis of the jaws [38]. The data is based on very few patients reported so far. One of them as reported by **Guhlmann *et al.* 1998** suffered from a secondary chronic osteomyelitis of the mandible.

Another case was of chronic paranasal sinusitis as reported by **Sugawara *et al.* 1998**. A report on osteomyelitis in head and neck and PET was published by **Hakim *et al.* in 2006**. He evaluated the value of 18FDG -PET *vs.* bone scintigraphy with 99mTc SPECT for primary diagnosis and follow-up in secondary chronic osteomyelitis of the mandible [49]. It was found that the scintigraphy was better for initial true-positive findings. On the contrary it was also evaluated that 18FDG-PET was much better for true-negative findings [8, 38]. The importance here lies in the early negative value of 18FDG-PET allowing the cessation of concomitant antibiotic therapy. Even if the results in this report do not confirm good accuracy and predictive value for osteomyelitis in the mandible compared with the rest of the body, further studies must be done. Without doubt, more data is needed to clearly elucidate the factors which favour the use of PET [8].

c) Combined Positron Emission Tomography/Computed Tomography Imaging

The fused PET/CT imaging is also known as hybrid imaging. It combines the advantages of a detailed imaging of the anatomy (with the help of CT) combined with detection of local metabolic activity pattern with the help of hybrid cameras to highlight the part of the body in which the radiopharmaceutical is administered.

Sometimes MRI scan can also be superimposed with PET scans instead of CT scans. Hence, this newer technique offers direct information of form and function of bone pathology simultaneously which would otherwise require an invasive procedure or may be rather impossible to achieve. Henceforth this particular procedure helps the physician to optimize initial therapy as well as follow-up. In comparison to CT and other conventional bone scans, PET/CT can even help to plan surgery with great precision that too in advance. Similarly in cases of primary chronic osteomyelitis, it is highly desirable to obtain a biopsy from a representative area with disease activity. These fusion images of the PET/CT scan of that area will be able to provide the clinician more precise map of the desired location. Possible combination with navigation systems will even increase the accuracy [8]. With the increasing availability and use of these combined PET/CT scanners, multimodality imaging (Nuclear Medicine/Radiology) will progress into clinical routine diagnostics, thus broadening expertise in diagnosing various pathologies including osteomyelitis of the jaws. Since this technique is quite advantageous, it is becoming more apparent amongst the clinicians and is on the verge of becoming the future gold standard technique in the diagnosis of osteomyelitis of the jaws.

E. Ultrasonography

There is vast literature which highlights the usage of ultrasonography (USG) in the diagnosis of osteomyelitis of jaws. According to **Nath *et al.* in 1992**, a sonographic diagnosis of osteomyelitis can be made if there is evidence of fluid present directly in contact with bone without any intervention of soft tissues.

Ultrasound (Fig. **5.8**) may also reveal elevation of the periosteum (by more than 2 mm) and thickening of the periosteum if the patient is suffering form osteomyelitis. Ultrasound may also improve the yield from fine needle biopsies as aspiration of the swelling can be planned guided by pus found in ultrasonography.

Advantages of Ultrasonography in the cases of Osteomyelitis of jaws (According to **Pineda *et al.* in 2009**) [38]:

a. It is readily accessible and can be performed quickly without delay.
b. It leads to minimal discomfort to the patient.
c. It is even found advantageous in regions which are complicated by orthopedic instrumentation which might not be well seen with MRI or CT.
d. It may prove to be useful in patients in whom MRI is contraindicated [38].
e. Lower cost.
f. It does not involve ionizing radiation.
g. It offers real time imaging.

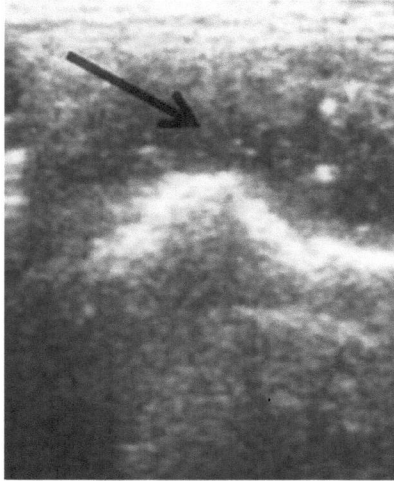

Fig. (5.8). Ultrasonography showing abscess surrounding the right condyle of mandible with erosions.

For these above mentioned reasons, ultrasonography is considered as a useful tool in the evaluation of musculoskeletal infections. It is found to be particularly helpful in differentiating acute or chronic infections from tumors or noninfective conditions [38].

According to **Cardinal** *et al.* **in 2001**, it is also able to localize the site and extent of infection, identify precipitating factors such as foreign bodies or fistulae, and provides guidance for diagnostic or therapeutic aspiration or biopsy [38]. **Pineda** *et al.* **in 2009** stated that ultrasonography (Fig. **5.8**) can detect features of osteomyelitis several days earlier as compared to conventional radiographs [38]. According to **Collado** *et al.* **in 2008**, ultrasonography is predominately more in helpful in case of children [48].

In the cases of acute osteomyelitis, ultrasonography may present with elevation of the periosteum by a hypoechoic layer of purulent material [38]. In chronic osteomyelitis, it can also be used to assess involvement of the adjacent soft tissues. Soft tissue abscesses related to chronic osteomyelitis are identified as [51] hypoechoic or anechoic fluid collections which may extend around the bony contours [38].

According to **Pineda in 2006**, cortical erosions can also become apparent on ultrasonography [38]. According to **Kaiser in 1994**, in pediatric patients, ultrasonography can spot osteomyelitis earlier as compared to plain radiographs. **Collado** *et al.* **in 2008** stated that in case of pediatric patients, joint effusion or subperiosteal fluid associated with osteomyelitis can be identified with the help of USG before it becomes apparent on plain radiographs [48, 49]. Since it is non-invasive and is dynamic, the added advantage is that it does not requires to sedate small children as there will be no blurring of the image or motion related artifacts.

Martinoli in 1998 stated the use of colour Doppler technique in osteomyelitis. **Collado *et al.* in 2008** stated that Power Doppler sonography significantly improves the sensitivity towards the detection of blood flow in the area concerned.

Color Doppler produces a picture of a blood vessel with the help of a computer programme. A computer converts the Doppler sounds into colours that are overlaid on the image of the blood vessel. This colour represents the speed and direction of blood flow through the vessel. Power Doppler on the other hand is a newer ultrasound technique which is almost 5 times more sensitive in detecting blood flow as compared to color Doppler. Power Doppler can get some images that are hard or impossible to get using standard color Doppler. But power Doppler is most commonly used to evaluate blood flow through vessels within solid organs. **Breidahl in 1996** advocated that Power Doppler sonography may be useful in recognizing infectious diseases [48]. **Newman in 1994** stated that Power Doppler sonography highlights hyperemia around the periosteum and surrounding soft tissue abscesses [48].

CHAPTER 6

Clinical and Radiological Features

Abstract: Thisis already discussed in the previous chapter that various classification systemsand nomenclatures of this disease have evolved with time. This is attributed to the fact that authors have classified osteomyelitis based on etiology, pathogenesis, clinical presentation, course, radiology, and histopathology. Osteomyelitis of the jaws presents with a varying clinical picture and henceforth it sometimes presents as a dilemmato the oral physician. This particular chapter highlights the various clinical *f*eatures of different types of osteomyelitis as projected by the researchers from time to time. This will help the students as well as researchers to derive the facts about the superimposingclinical features of the types of osteomyelitis classified separately as wellas different clinical presentation of similar type of osteomyelitis highlighted by different authors in the literature.

Keywords: Acute Suppurative Osteomyelitis, Adult Onset Primary Chronic Osteomyeiltis, Clinical features of Osteomyelitis of jaws, Early Onset Primary Chronic Osteomyelitis, Infantile .osteomyelitis, Non-suppurative osteomyelitis, Primary Chronic Osteomyelitis, Secondary Chronic Osteomyelitis, Sub acute stage of Osteomyelitis, SAPHO syndrome, Zurich Classification of Osteomyelitis.

A. ACUTE OSTEOMYELITIS

Literature reveals that four types of Osteomyelitis of the jaws are observed clinically [1]

1. **Acute Suppurative**
2. **Secondary Chronic**, a form that begins as acute Osteomyelitis and becomes chronic
3. **Primary Chronic**, a form that has manifested no acute phase previously, having always been a low grade infection
4. **Non Suppurative osteomyelitis**

A **sub acute stage** also exists in which acute symptoms such as elevated temperature and white blood cell count are nearly normal but the production of pus and extension into the adjacent bone continues [1]. It is not clearly defined in the literature.

According to **Schmidt and Townsend in 2008**, sub acute osteomyelitis describes a condition somewhat in between acute and chronic osteomyelitis with relatively moderate symptoms [33]. To avoid confusion and keep the classification simple, this term has been abandoned in the Zurich classification [8].

According to **Baltenspenger** in **Zurich classification in 2003**, acute and secondary chronic osteomyelitis are suppurative infections, whereas primary chronic osteomyelitis is, by definition, a nonsuppurative bone disease.

As mentioned previously, various classification systems and nomenclatures of this disease have evolved with time. The heterogeneity of the classification systems is borne by the fact that several modalities are used to describe and define maxillofacial osteomyelitis. These modalities include etiology and pathogenesis, clinical presentation, course, radiology, and histopathology.

According to **Lee in 2004 and Suei** *et al.* **in 2005**, the classification of mandibular osteomyelitis was found to be inconsistent and differed amongst references [22,34]. Furthermore, these classification forms represent a mixture of these criteria, causing confusion, thereby hindering student training and designing clinical research [8,34].

In **1991, Marx and Mercuri** were the first and only authors to define the duration for an acute osteomyelitis until it should be considered as chronic. They set an arbitrary time limit of 4 weeks after onset of disease. Pathological–anatomical onset of osteomyelitis corresponds to deep bacterial invasion into the medullar and cortical bone. After the period of 4 weeks, a persisting bone infection should be considered as secondary chronic osteomyelitis as shown in Fig. (**6.1**). Because of its simplicity and clarity, this criterion is also used in the Zurich classification to differentiate acute osteomyelitis from secondary chronic osteomyelitis cases [8].

DEMOGRAPHICS
(Acute and Secondary Chronic Osteomyelitis)

Acute and secondary chronic osteomyelitis may affect all ages and both sexes. There is a male predominance with a 2:1 ratio according to **Baltensperger in 2003**.

Further, **Koorbush** *et al.* **in 1992** described a male to female ratio of 3:1 in a survey of 35 patients.

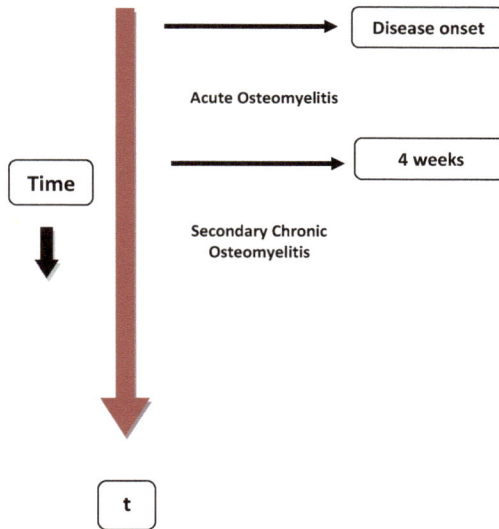

Fig. (6.1). Definition of acute and secondary chronic osteomyelitis of the jawbone (Adapted from Marx and Mercuri 1991).

An equal gender distribution was noted by **Daramola *et al*. in 1982** in a larger African patient population.

The mean age of onset of disease as described by **Baltensperger in 2003** is almost the same in cases of acute and secondary chronic osteomyelitis: 42.9 years (range 1–81 years) and 44.1 years (range 6–89 years) respectively.

In a retrospective analysis carried out by **Uche *et al*. in 2009**, the mean age of onset was found to be 58.3 years [35].

Acute Osteomyelitis

Depending on the intensity of the disease and the magnitude of imbalance between the host and the microbiological aggressors, three principal types of clinical courses of acute osteomyelitis can be distinguished [8]. It may be Acute suppurative, Subacute suppurative or clinically silent with or without suppuration.

Acute Suppurative Osteomyelitis

Synonyms:
Acute osteomyelitis, pyogenic osteomyelitis, subacute suppurative osteomyelitis.

According to **Caldwell in 1909**, it exists when an acute inflammatory process spreads through the medullary spaces of the bone with subsequent necrosis of variable amount of bone and there has been insufficient time for the body to react to the presence of the inflammatory infiltrate [13,50].

Incidence:
Patient of all ages can be affected by Osteomyelitis [50]. There is strong male predominance, approaching 75% in some reviews. Most cases involve the mandible.

According to **Adekeye *et al*. in 1975 and 1985**, maxillary disease becomes important primarily in pediatric patients [9] and in cases that arise from ANUG or NOMA in Nigerian populations [9, 13].

Adekeye *et al*. in 1985 also stated that these periodontal diseases cannot entirely explain the high incidence of osteomyelitis in maxilla as ANUG never led to osteomyelitis of the maxilla in Europe and North America [9]. In the maxilla the disease usually remains fairly localized to the area of initial infection. In the mandible the bone involvement tends to be more diffuse and widespread.

Microbiology:
It is usually a polymicrobial infection. Different types of organisms can be cultured from these lesions. According to **Fenner in 1932,** the most common are *Staphylococcus aureus* and Staphylococcus albus and various Streptococci. Anaerobes such as Bacteriodes, Porphyromonas, or Prevotella species also predominate [35].Vincent's spirochetes and Gram-negative bacilli may also be present [16].

Early Acute Suppurative Osteomyelitis

Clinical Features

Early cases (Figs. **6.2**, **6.3**) are characterized by [16]:

1. Generalized constitutional symptoms such as high intermittent fever, malaise, nausea, vomiting and anorexia. This was advocated by **Bitting and Durham in 1929**.
2. Deep seated boring, continuous intense pain in the affected area.
3. Intermittent paresthesia or anesthesia of the lower lip, which helps the clinician to distinguish this from alveolar abscess.
4. Facial cellulitis, or indurated swelling of moderate size, which is more confined to the periosteal envelop and its contents:
   i. Thrombosis of the inferior alveolar vasa nervorum.
   ii. Rise in pressure from edema in the inferior alveolar canal. This was inferred by **Oechsner in 1914.**

iii. Teeth are mobile and tender to percussion.
5. It can be characterized by trismus in children which is:
    i. Fulminating and involves of the maxilla or mandible.
    ii. Severe and serious.
    iii. Complicated by the presence of unerupted developing tooth buds, which become necrotic and act as foreign bodies and prolong the disease process.

Long-term involvement of the Temporomandibular joint (TMJ) can cause ankylosis of TMJ and subsequently affect the growth and development of facial structures.

According to **Fenner in 1932,** a clearly identifiable cause, usually deep caries in an involved tooth is one of the factors which may point towards acute osteomyelitis (Fig. **6.2**). Additionally, positive bone scan finding is indicative of acute osteomyelitis. It has a rapid onset and course. At this stage the process is truly intramedullary, the teeth are not mobile and fistulae are not present [51, 52].

According to **Caldwell in 1909,** such cases present with mild leukocytosis (PMNL).

According to **Bitting in 1929,** laboratory studies show mild leukocytosis (PMNL) along with albuminuria [16].

Established Suppurative Osteomyelitis [51]

In adults, it is more common in the mandible and involves alveolar process, angle of the mandible, posterior part of the ramus and the coronoid process.

Linsey in 1953 advocated the rarity of osteomyelitis of the condyle [16].

Established Cases (Fig. 6.3) are Characterized by [16]

1. Deep pain, malaise, fever, dehydration, anorexia.
2. Teeth in the involved area begin to loosen and become sensitive to percussion.
3. Purulent discharge through sinuses which may occur:
    a. Intraorally around the gingival sulcus or through the buccal vestibule
    b. Extraorally on the face, through the cutaneous fistulae.
4. Fetid odour is often present.
5. Trismus and regional lymphadenopathy is present.
6. Dehydration, acidosis and toxemia. This was stated by **Bitting in 1929**.

Diagnosis of Acute Osteomyelitis [54]

• Pus on aspiration.

- Positive bacterial culture from bone or blood.
- Presence of classic signs and symptoms of acute Osteomyelitis.
- Radiographic changes typical of Osteomyelitis (Fig. **6.3**).

According to **Saraswathi** *et al.* **in 2002,** two of the above listed findings must be present to achieve the diagnosis of acute osteomyelitis [54].

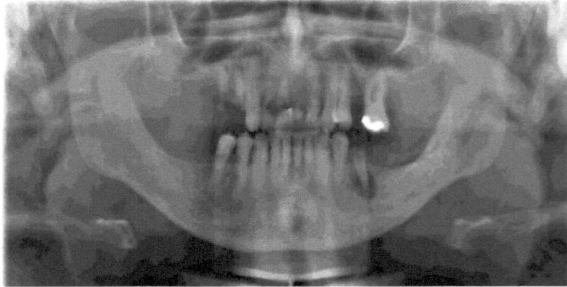

Fig. (6.2). Osteomyelitis of left side of the mandible (Courtsey: Dr. John KM Aps).

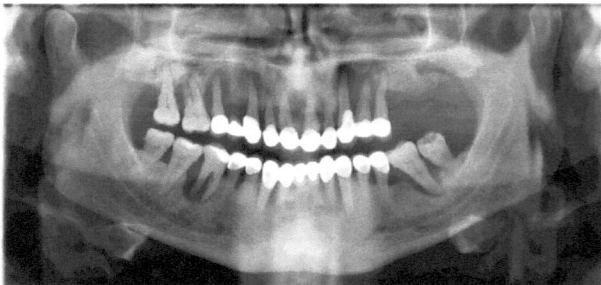

Fig. (6.3). Osteomyelitis of the maxilla bilaterally in the canine and premolar region with altered trabecular pattern (Courtesy: Dr. John KM Aps).

Laboratory Studies Show [16]

   i. Leukocytosis according to **Oechsner in 1914** (PMNL) [55 - 59].
  ii. Elevated Erythrocytic Sedimentation Rate (ESR).
 iii. Anemia.
 iv. Albuminuria [16].

Blood cultures, wound culture & sensitivity, and complete blood count along with peaks and troughs on any antimicrobial prescribed should be assessed on a regular basis.

Roentgenographic Features

Bitting & Durham in 1929 stated that no radiographic changes may be identifiable in very early stage of the disease [26,55,57,59].

Aliabadi & Nikpoor in 1994 stated that the bone may be filled with inflammatory cells and may show no radiographic changes until the disease has developed for at least one or two weeks [26,53]. At this time diffuse lytic changes in the bone begin to appear. Individual trabeculae become fuzzy and indistinct and radiolucent areas begin to appear. These have ill defined margins and have a moth eaten appearance [50].

Coviello in 2007 stated that conventional radiographs do not show changes early on the disease process [30], but strongly positive radionucleotide scan results together with these clinical findings strongly support the diagnosis of acute suppurative intramedullary osteomyelitis.

Periphery

Acute Osteomyelitis most often presents an ill defined periphery with a gradual transition to normal trabeculae [53]. In some cases there is saucer shaped area of destruction with irregular margin and containing teeth with variable amount of supporting bone [51].

Internal Structure

The first radiographic evidence of acute Osteomyelitis is a slight decrease in the density of the involved bone with thinning and loss of sharpness of the existing trabeculae (Figs. **6.2**, **6.3** and **6.4**) [53]. The trabeculae soon loose their continuity as well as density. Individual trabeculae become fuzzy and indistinct [51]. In time the bone destruction becomes more profound, resulting in an area of radiolucency in one focal area or in scattered regions throughout the involved bone. Later, the appearance of sclerotic regions becomes apparent.

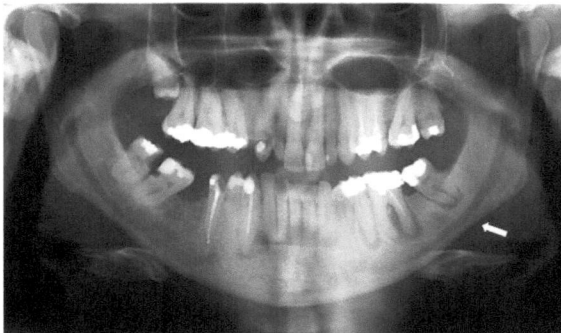

Fig. (6.4). Osteomyelitis of the left side of the mandible in the ramus with fuzzy trabecular pattern (Courtesy Dr. John KM Aps).

Sequestra may be present (Fig. **6.5**) but usually are more numerous in chronic forms. Sequestra can be identified by closely inspecting a region of bone destruction (radiolucency) for an island of bone. This island of nonvital bone may vary in size from a small dot (smaller sequestra usually seen in young patients) to large fragments of radiopaque bone [53].

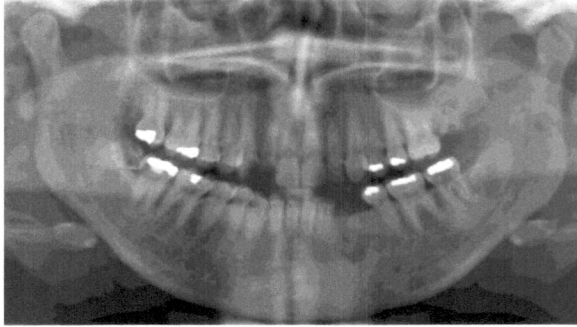

Fig. (6.5). Osteomyelitis of the left mandible in the canine region with sequester formation (Courtesy Dr. John KM Aps).

Effect on the Surrounding Structures [53]

Acute Osteomyelitis can stimulate either bone resorption or bone formation. Portions of the cortical bone may be resorbed. An inflammatory exudate can lift the periosteum and stimulate bone formation. Radiographically this appears as a thin, faint radiopaque line adjacent and almost parallel or slightly convex to the surface of the bone. A radiolucent band separates this periosteal new bone from the bone surface.

Lamina Dura [51]

There is loss of continuity of the lamina dura, which is seen in more than one tooth.

Histologic Features [1]

The marrow is infiltrated by polymorphonuclear leukocytes [55], lymphocytes and plasma cells. Necrotic bone devoid of osteocytes from the lacunae and areas of scalloped resorption are usually present. Regions of distinct bone sclerosis, reactive bone formation demonstrating plump and active osteoblasts, obliterative endarteritis and thrombosis may be seen. Varying degrees of interstitial tissue, oedema and peripheral fibrovasascular stromal connective tissue are frequently present. Active osteoclastic resorption of bone may be noted in more peripheral portions.

Differential Diagnosis [53]

The differential diagnosis of acute Osteomyelitis includes

a. Fibrous dysplasia seen especially in children

According to **Sheikh and Pallagatti in 2010,** it is difficult to differentiate between osteomyelitis and fibrous dysplasia is difficult when there is no trauma and no systemic disease [60]. The clinical findings in fibrous dysplasia show asymptomatic enlargement of the involved bone leading to facial asymmetry.

According to **Sheikh and Pallagatti in 2010**, the most useful radiographic characteristics to distinguish Osteomyelitis from fibrous dysplasia is the way the enlargement of bone occurs [60]. The new bone that enlarges the jaws in Osteomyelitis is laid down by the periosteum and therefore is on the outside of the outer cortical plate. In fibrous dysplasia the new bone is produced on the inner side of the mandible (Fig. **6.6**). Thus the cortex, which may be thinned, is on the outside and contains the lesion. This point of differentiation is important because the histologic appearance of a biopsy of a new periosteal bone in Osteomyelitis may be similar to that of fibrous dysplasia, and the condition may be reported as such.

According to **Petrikowski *et al.* in 1995**, fibrous dysplasia is more commonly granular and exhibits a fingerprint bone pattern which is a useful distinguishing feature from osteomyelitis. Furthermore superior displacement of mandibular canal strongly suggests a diagnosis of fibrous dysplasia and is a unique characteristic which is not seen in osteomyelitis [61].

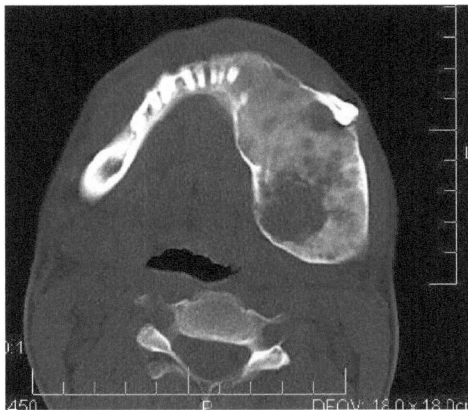

Fig. (6.6). An Axial CT scan of a patient with Fibrous Dysplasia with expansion of the left mandibular body. The cortex is seen on the periphery of the enlargement.

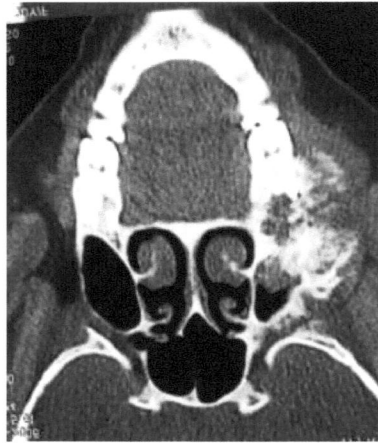

Fig. (6.7). Axial CT of a case of maxillary osteosarcoma with soft tissue window. There is infiltration of the buccal soft tissues with destruction of the walls of maxillary sinus with sunray type of ossification.

b. Malignant neoplasia

According to **Sheikh and Pallagatti in 2010**, malignant neoplastic diseases like osteosarcoma [60] and squamous cell carcinoma that invade the mandible may be difficult to differentiate from acute osteomyelitis. If part of the inflammatory periosteal bone has been destroyed, the possibility of the malignant neoplasm should be considered (Fig. **6.7**) [61].

c. Other bony destructive lesions of the jaw

The differential diagnosis may include other lesions that can cause bone destruction and may stimulate periosteal bone reaction. This is similar to that seen in inflammatory lesions.

Langerhans cell histiocytosis causes lytic ill-defined bone destruction and often results in the formation of periosteal reactive bone formation. This lesion rarely simulates a sclerotic bone reaction such as that seen in Osteomyelitis. Leukemia and lymphoma may stimulate a similar periosteal reaction.

Infantile Osteomyelitis [16, 51]

It is a particular form of acute osteomyelitis, referred to as neonatal osteomyelitis in infants and young children. It is a well recognized entity that is becoming uncommon nowadays because of antibiotic drugs and sophistication of medical and dental practice.

Synonyms: Osteomyelitis maxillaries neonaturum, maxillitis of infancy.

It is a rare type of osteomyelitis seen in infants involving the maxilla. **Wilensky in 1932 [16]** described osteomyelitis in infants in a comprehensive manner.

The condition was first described by **Rees in 1847**. According to **McCash in 1953**, less than one hundred cases have been reported in the English and American literature.

According to **McCash in 1953**, reference has been found to only thirteen cases since the introduction of penicillin [12].

Asherson in 1939, in a comprehensive review, stated that he saw only four cases during ten years work at two London hospitals [12].

Lacy and Engel in 1939 reported one case and summarised thirty-six cases reported between 1922 and 1939 [12]. Further many cases have also been reported by **Hitchin and Naylor in 1957 [12]**. Subsequently, cases have been reported by **Norgaard & Pindborg in 1959** and **Cavanagh in 1960 [12,16]**.

This condition deserves special mention because of its seriousness and potential for facial deformities resulting from delayed or inappropriate treatment.

Etiology

1. **Trauma**: The access may be through a break in the mucosa due to trauma such as perinatal trauma caused to oral mucosa during delivery or when the obstetrician's finger is inserted into the child's mouth. Other traumatic causes include injury to the mucosa caused by mucous suction bulb used to clear the airway soon after birth.
2. **Infection of the maxillary sinus:** This was advocated by **Macbeth in 1951** to be a causative factor [9].
3. **Contaminated human or artificial nipples**
4. **Infections from the nose:** This was proposed by **Paunz** in **1926** and **Ramon** *et al.* in **1977 [16]**.
5. **Hematogenous invasion by streptococci and pneumococci:** This was also reported by **Wilensky in 1932 [9]**.

Clinical Features

According to **McCash in 1953**, it is seen a few weeks after birth. The disease shows considerable variation in severity. It is of a sudden onset and acute course. The disease may also have slow onset and a chronic course. In the acute stage, there is severe pain and high fever [12].

With chronic course of the disease, there is moderate pain and slight fever.

a. **General body manifestations**: Pyrexia, anorexia, dehydration, convulsions, or vomiting.
b. **Extraoral examination**: Facial cellulitis seen centered around the orbit, inner canthal swelling, palpebral edema, closure of the eye, conjunctivitis, and proptosis.
c. **Intra oral examination:**
   i. The maxilla is usually affected, especially the molar region.
   ii. Sub periosteal abscesses in alveolar region. These are seen as buccal or palatal swellings.
   iii. Fluctuation is often present.
   iv. Fistulae or pus draining tracts may exist in alveolar mucosa.
d. **Laboratory findings**: Leukocytosis is generally present.
e. **Microbiology**: Organisms implicated are *Staphylococcus aureus* and Streptococci.
f. **Radiological findings**: In the early stage, the radiographs are of little value, as there is minimal bone involvement. In later stages, intraoral films help to locate sequestra and necrotic tooth germs.
g. **Risks**: Prior to the antibiotic era, mortality and morbidity was very high. With the advent of the antibiotics, it is considerably reduced. Death usually occurs due to the spread of the infection to the brain (cavernous sinus thrombophlebitis).

Instances of extension into the dural sinuses have also been reported. According to **McCash in 1953,** the risks involved are

  i. Permanent optic damage
 ii. Neurological complications
iii. Loss of tooth buds and bone.

Differential Diagnosis

1. Dacrocystitis neonatorum
2. Orbital cellulitis
3. Ophthalmia neonaturum
4. Infantile cortical hyperostosis

The oral manifestations can help to distinguish infantile osteomyelitis from these above mentioned conditions.

B. SECONDARY CHRONIC OSTEOMYELITIS

The term "Secondary Chronic Osteomyelitis" (SCO) have been used by **Hjorting-Hansen in 1970, Panders & Hadders in 1970** and **Schelhorn & Zenk** in **1989** from Europe. It was used interchangeably with chronic suppurative osteomyelitis in Anglo-American texts by **Marx in 1991**. **Bernier** *et al.* used this term in **1995** and **Topazian** used it in **1994 & 2002** [8].

It is considered as a sequel of Acute Osteomyelitis. Its clinical presentation may also vary depending upon the intensity of the disease as well as on the magnitude of imbalance between the host defence system, microbiological aggressors and time [8].

Clinical Features

Clinically the patient with SCO may present with pain and swelling which are usually less extensive as compared to the acute stage (Fig. **6.8**). Acute stage presents with deep and intense pain while the chronic stage presents with a more dull pain. Painful swelling caused by local edema and abscess formation in the acute stage is subsided and it is replaced by a harder and palpable tenderness caused due to periosteal reaction [8].

According to **Leroy in 1986** [63], the patients with SCO will present with sequester and fistula formation. These are regarded as classical signs of secondary chronic osteomyelitis. Further such patients can often present with fetid odour. However the presence of fetid odour is less frequent than in cases of acute abscess formation.

Patients may also present with disturbed occlusion. This may be attributed to the fact that the process of osteomyelitis may lead to raise in intraosseous pressure which in turn can lead to elongation and mobility of the tooth [73] (Fig. **6.9**).

According to **Bernhard** *et al.* **in 1997**, there are cases of SCO in which the acute phase is not evident. In other words these are the cases with silent acute phase. In such cases, the secondary chronic osteomyelitis will not present any specific clinical signs and symptoms [62]. Cause of infection in such cases is considered to be a low-grade infection. These low grade infections cannot be even fully eradicated by host defences. These cases of SCO will present with less pus, fistula, and sequester formation as compared to usual cases. Since these are the distinguishing features of SCO, these cases may even lack these symptoms at progressive phases of the disease. Radiologically these cases may present with a diffuse sclerosis with little to no osteolysis (Fig. **6.9**).

Literature reveals that tentatively a number of reported cases of Diffuse Sclerosing Osteomyelitis (DSO) actually fall into this category. Henceforth in such cases it is very difficult to differentiate them from primary chronic osteomyelitis [8]. So to attain pertinent diagnosis, the course of the disease must be reviewed thoroughly in collaboration with different imaging modalities.

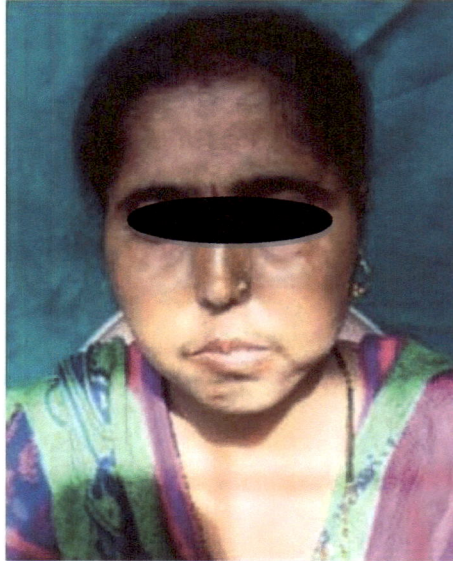

Fig. (6.8). Profile of a patient presenting with swelling and dull pain in the left side of the face with numbness of the left lower lip.

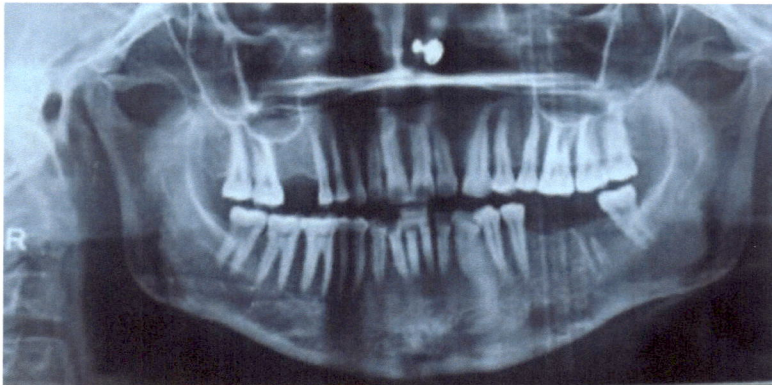

Fig. (6.9). OPG revealing destruction of bone in the left mandibular body with evidence of Extraction socket with respect to 36,37.

Radiological Features

According to **Klinefelter in 1926**, untreated or insufficiently treated cases of acute osteomyelitis of the jaws may progress to chronic osteomyelitis [63,64]. **LeRoy in 1986** also supported the above findings. It is referred to as SCO in these cases. It designates persistent infection of the osseous structures of the jaw exceeding a time frame of 4 weeks [8].

Conventional Radiological Signs

According to **Baltensperger in 2003**, the panoramic view is considered as a standard examination so as to assess the osseous situation as well as the status of the dentition [8]. Secondary chronic osteomyelitis affecting the mandible is much better recognized as compared to the upper jaw (Fig. **6.9**).

According to **Bernhard *et al.* in 1997**, conventional radiological signs seen in the case of secondary chronic osteomyelitis of the jaws may include the following [62]:

a. Areas of increased radiopacity with loss of bone trabeculae.
b. Minor areas of radiolucency with interruption of cortical bone (Fig. **6.9**)
c. Sequester formation
d. Calcified periosteal reaction
e. Pathological fracture

According to **LeRoy in 1986**, sequester formation can be seen by conventional radiographs (Figs. **6.10** and **6.11**) in cases of Secondary chronic osteomyelitis [63].

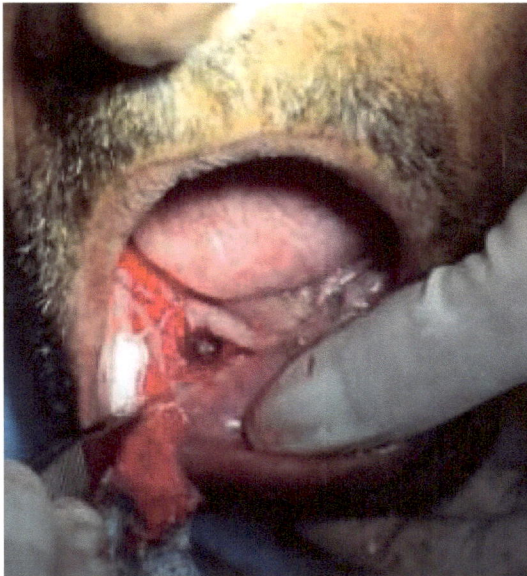

Figs. (6.10). Clinical presentation of a patient with Sequester formation.

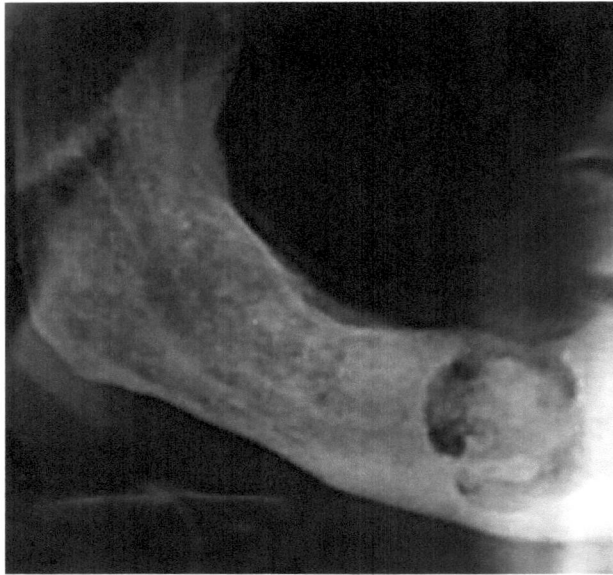

Figs. (6.11). Radiological presentation of a patient with Sequester formation.

According to **Taori in 2005**, CT scan is the standard imaging modality for evaluating the bone for sequestrum formation [65].

The signs in Computed Tomography in secondary chronic osteomyelitis of the jaws are as follows:

a. According to **Bernhard *et al.* in 1997,** areas of increased bone density *i.e.* cancellous bone sclerosis and trabecular & cortical bone thickening by endosteal or periosteal apposition are the cardinal CT changes indicating secondary osteomyelitis of the jaws [62].

b. Calcified linear periosteal reaction as dictated by **Bernhard *et al.* in1997** [62].

c. Areas of mixed sclerosis. According to **Schuknecht *et al.* in 1997** and **Seabolt *et al.* in 1995**, these areas of sclerosis may be accompanied by gross sequester formation and cortical erosion.

d. Pathological fracture (Fig. **6.12**). According to **Orpe *et al.* in 1996**, the availability of CT has tremendously improved the sequestra detection from 45% on the plain films to 91% [8]. Further CT also helps to precisely depict the bucco-lingual positioning of the sequester inside the jaws.

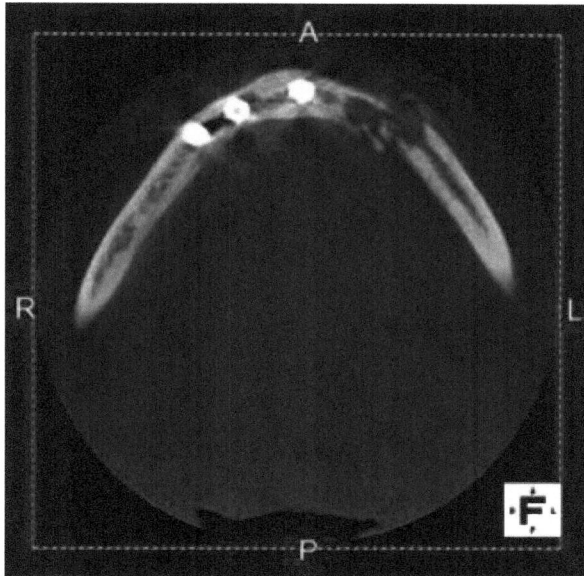

Fig. (6.12). Cone beam Computed tomography scans (axial view) demonstrate massive destruction of the left mandible with significant osteolysis and sequester formation. A strong periosteal reaction on the buccal aspect of the mandible is evident with formation of a neocortex. **(Courtsey: Dr. Maria Vascenclos)**.

According to Schuknecht in 2009, SCO may present with the following signs in Magnetic Resonance Imaging:

a. Marrow fat is replaced by low signal tissue with increase in T2 signal intensity because of presence of oedema.
b. T1 contrast enhancement due to major inflammation.
c. There is marrow space enlargement with loss or thinning of cortical plate.
d. Periosteal extension of inflammatory tissue leading to contrast enhancing periosteal reaction.
e. Soft tissue contrast enhancement.

Laboratory Findings

Laboratory findings are of a little or sometimes no diagnostic value in cases of secondary chronic osteomyelitis of jaws. It is so because laboratory findings in SCO of the jaws are less prominent as compared to acute osteomyelitis. This highlights that there is localized form of infectious process in SCO leading to moderate systemic reactions. This is especially true in cases with little or mild clinical symptoms where laboratory findings can be almost normal. Microbiologically, according to **Leroy in 1986**, chronic osteomyelitis reflects normal oral flora, *Staphylococcus aureus* and aerobic gram negative rods [63].

Histopathological Findings

There are large amounts of polymorphonuclear leucocytes, macrophages, and plasma cells, accompanied by a variable degree of marrow fibrosis and reactive bone formation. In cases with a less fulminate course (*e.g.*, more chronic), marrow fibrosis and reactive bone scleroses are predominant. In some instances, according to **Montonen in 1993**, if there is proper staining and magnification, bacteria may be identified on histopathological specimens [66]. In cases of secondary chronic osteomyelitis of the jaws caused by Actinomyces, "drusen" formation can be observed, which is classical for this type of infection.

Differential Diagnosis

Early-stage secondary chronic osteomyelitis (predominant osteolysis)	Advanced-stage secondary chronic osteomyelitis (osteolysis and sclerosis)
a) Primary bone tumors [64]	a) Primary bone tumors
b) Bone metastasis	b) Bone metastasis
c) Primary intraosseous or invasive growing squamous cell carcinoma	c) Primary intraosseous or invasive growing squamous cell carcinoma
d) Early osteoradionecrosis	d) Osteoradionecrosis
e) Eosinophilic granuloma	e) Osteochemonecrosis (bisphosphonate induced)
f) Plasmocytoma	f) Plasmocytoma
g) Demineralized bone in dialysis patients	g) Demineralized bone in dialysis patients
	h) Tendoperiostitis
	i) Primary chronic osteomyelitis

C. PRIMARY CHRONIC OSTEOMYELITIS

The term "primary chronic osteomyelitis," was used by **Spiessl in 1959**. **Hjørting-Hansen** used this term in **1970** for a rare inflammatory disease having unknown etiology [8,67]. This term was also used in the Zurich system of classification of osteomyelitis of the jaws in 2003 and was also considered to be of unknown etiology [8,67]. According to **Baltensperger *et al.* in 2004** it is a rare, strictly nonsuppurative chronic inflammation of the jaw bone [67].

According to **Bevin *et al.* in 2008**, it is considered as a rare disease with chronic inflammation of the jaw bone. It is not associated with any pus formation, sinus formation or sequestration [67,68].

Paula *et al.* in 2009 advocated the use of other terms like Diffuse Sclerosing Osteomyelitis (DSO) of the jaw, Chronic Recurrent Multifocal Osteomyelitis (CRMO), or SAPHO (Synovitis, Acne, Pustulosis, Hyperostosis, and Osteitis) syndrome [67,68] for primary chronic osteomyelitis (PCO).

Suei *et al.* in 1995 used the term DSO or CRMO for Primary chronic osteomyelitis [68].

Kahn *et al.* in 1994 used the term SAPHO syndrome for PCO [69,70].

According to **Bevin *et al.* in 2008**, 'primary chronic osteomyelitis' infers to the patient who has never undergone any appreciable acute phase of the disease. Further such patients lack a definitive initiating event and follows an insidious course [8,68].

Incidence

As stated by **Baltensperger in 2004**, primary chronic osteomyelitis (PCO) of the jaw is not a well described disease entity [67]. **Jacobsson in 1984** and **Van Merkestyn *et al.* in 1988** confirmed that it occurred mostly in adults. **Montonen *et al.* in 1993** also defined its existence mostly in adults, which was in accordance to the previous authors [67]. However, **Paula *et al.* in 2009** stated that it can be found in all age groups [69].

Literature reveals that PCO is very rarely reported in children and adolescents. However authors like **Panders and Hadders** in 1970, **Ellis *et al.*** in 1977, **Eisenbud *et al.*** in 1981, **Mattison *et al.*** in 1981, **Nortje *et al.*** in 1988, **Betts *et al.*** in 1996 and **Heggie in 2000** have presented single case reports of PCO in this age group [67].

Baltenspenger in 2004 first described the age-related prevalence of Primary Chronic Osteomyelitis [67]. According to him the initial peak onset of the disease is in adolescence, between 11 and 20 years, and a second peak, after age of 50 years [67]. The second peak was documented to be less prominent. According to **Paula *et al.* in 2009**, it has a 2:1 predilection for women [69 - 71].

Etiology

According to **Bevin *et al.* in 2008**, the etiology of PCO is unknown and theories include bacterial infection (dental or bacteremia from distant foci), vascular deficiency (localized endarteritis), or autoimmune disease [68] as various etiological factors. Even though some authors like **Marx in 1994** and **Jacobsson in 1982**, suggest primary chronic osteomyelitis to be infectious in origin [69, 71], however there is a negative response to antibiotic treatment in such cases [69]. **Baltensperger in 2004** stated that it is a disease of unknown etiology [8,67,81].

Clinical Features

The clinical features of PCO are mild as compared to other acute and/or chronic suppurative infections [81 - 84]. Hence they are not much disturbing and painful.

Most of the cases of primary chronic osteomyelitis feature periodic episodes of onset that too with varying intensity [8,67]. The duration of these episodes is documented to last from a few days to several weeks [67]. These episodes are also marked by certain periods of silence where the patient may experience little to no clinical symptoms [8,67].

According to **Paula *et al.* in 2009**, the active periods of the disease are marked by pain which is dull to severe along with limited jaw movements associated with myofascial pain [69]. Variable swelling can also be observed [69]. It can also be associated with regional lymphadenopathy and paresthesia in the region supplied by inferior alveolar nerve [8]. The reduced sensation of the inferior alveolar nerve is known as Vincent's symptom.

According to **Baltensperger in 2004** and **Paula *et al.* in 2009**, primary chronic osteomyelitis of the jaws mostly targets the mandible. **Flygare *et al.* in 1997** reported a unique case of primary chronic osteomyelitis which presented with the involvement of both jaws [8].

Since this disease is insidious in nature, it is sometimes difficult to differentiate this disease from certain kind of malignancies (osteosarcoma, chondrosarcoma, Ewing's sarcoma) as well as benign conditions (fibrous dysplasia, ossifying/non-ossifying fibroma)especially in children as well as adolescents who particularly present with mandibular enlargements [67].

Sub-classification of Primary Chronic Osteomyelitis of the Jaws

As stated earlier, according to **Baltensperger in 2003** and **Baltensperger *et al.* in 2004**, the onset of PCO revealed two incidence peaks. The initial peak was in adolescents of 11-20 years while less prominent second peak was after the age of 50 years.

A closer analysis of Primary Chronic Osteomyelitis was performed by **Baltenspenger *et al.* in 2004** regarding the clinical, radiological and histopathological features of the disease which revealed few differences in these features on the basis of age of onset of the disease.

On the basis of these differences, **Baltensperger *et al.* in 2004** subclassified PCO as follows [8]:

  i. Early-onset primary chronic osteomyelitis
 ii. Adult-onset primary chronic osteomyelitis

Few patients with PCO of the jaws may present osteomyelitic lesions in the other parts of the skeleton as well. Such patients may or may not present additional symptoms in skin or other joints in the body. Jaw involvement in such patients is considered as a part of syndrome and therefore is described as syndrome-associated primary chronic osteomyelitis of the jaw.

The term Diffuse Sclerosing Osteomyelitis (DSO) is also used synonymously with PCO in the literature. Several authors also reveal that this term is predominantly used in English Literature and is a broad non-specific term which is used to describe different disease processes [67]. However according to **Baltenspenger** *et al.* **in 2004**, DSO is strictly radiological representation of the disease [67].

According to **Hjørting-Hansen in 1970, Ellis** *et al.* **in 1977, Eisenbud** *et al.* **in 1981**, and **Eyrich** *et al.* **in 1999**, such radiological appearances can be caused by several similar processes including primary or secondary chronic osteomyelitis, chronic tendoperiostitis, ossifying periostitis or Garre's osteomyelitis [67]. So the term Diffuse Sclerosing Osteomyelitis is mostly used as a synonym for PCO [21].

Adult-Onset Primary Chronic Osteomyelitis

It describes cases with an onset of symptoms in the adult patient after 20-years of age. The clinical symptoms include chronic inflammation of the jawbone with swelling and pain, ranging from dull to sharp, without signs of suppuration. Intensity of the symptoms decreases as the disease progresses [8].

Several authors believe PCO to be infectious in origin. Hence according to them, it is believed to be a chronic infection which is actually still unproven. However **Jacobson** *et al.* **in 1982** and **Marx** *et al.* **in 1994** identified Propionibacterium acne, species of Actinomyces, and Eikenella corrodens in patients with primary chronic osteomyelitis, still they cannot be considered as a proof of infectious hypothesis. This was attributed to methodological deficits in these studies with possible contamination of the specimens. [8].

Immunological parameters reveal a mild elevation of the erythrocyte sedimentation rate and the C-reactive protein level. These findings are usually accompanied by a normal leukocyte count. During onset and active periods of the disease, subfebrile body temperatures can also be noted. According to **Baltensperger in 2003** and **Baltensperger** *et al.* **in 2004**, body temperature was found to be normal in less active or silent periods of primary chronic osteomyelitis.

According to **Jacobson** *et al.* **in 1982**, the patients of PCO of jaws may present with hyperactivity, hypoactivity, and even total impairment of immune response. An alteration in these basic immunological parameters reflecting the clinical course seems reasonable [8, 84]. These observations were further confirmed by **Eyrich** *et al.* **in 1999**.

Early-onset Primary Chronic Osteomyelitis (Juvenile Chronic Osteomyelitis)

Early-onset Primary Chronic Osteomyelitis describes cases with an onset in childhood or adolescence. According to **Eyrich** *et al.* **in 2003** and **Bevin in 2008**, PCO when occurs in children and adolescents is known as Garre's osteomyelitis [67,68].

In recent publications done by **Eyrich** *et al.* **in 1999** and **2003**, early-onset Primary Chronic Osteomyelitis is also known by the term "juvenile chronic osteomyelitis". **Baltensperger** *et al.* **in 2004** also used this same term. This term was also used by **Heggie and co-workers in 2000 and 2003** to describe their young patients with primary chronic osteomyelitis affecting the jaws. The clinical symptoms of early-onset primary chronic osteomyelitis are generally the same as in adults but usually of stronger intensity.

Jacobson in 1984 and **Eyrich** *et al.* **in 2003** stated that in the active periods of the disease, there is more extensive periosteal reaction.

Baltensperger in 2003 and **Baltensperger** *et al.* **in 2004** stated that the active period of the disease is marked by a more prominent swelling as well as tenderness of the jaw owing to the extensive periosteal reaction in such cases. Hence, the swelling leads to expansion of the mandibular bone with a pseudotumor-like appearance. Radiologically this pseudotumor presents with a mixed pattern of regions of osteolysis embedded in pronounced sclerotic bone. The anatomical architecture is destructed due to periosteal reaction and there is formation of an appearance of onion peel as seen in cases of ossifying periostitis.

According to **Sheikh and Pallagatti in 2010**, this may resemble Osteosarcoma or other bone malignancies [60]. **Sheikh** *et al.* **in 2010** further stated that malignancy can be ruled out with the help of biopsy in such instances [60].

It is of interest to know the variability of the clinical course of early-onset primary chronic osteomyelitis (Fig. **6.13**). It shows high variability from patient to patient. Since the disease process is active during puberty, the intensity of such cases decreases as the patient outgrows puberty. However, literature has also evidence of continuation of the disease process up to adulthood despite of therapeutic interventions [8]. Literature further revels lack of data on this rare disease. Hence it is not possible to validate the clinical course and outcome of this disease in a given patient.

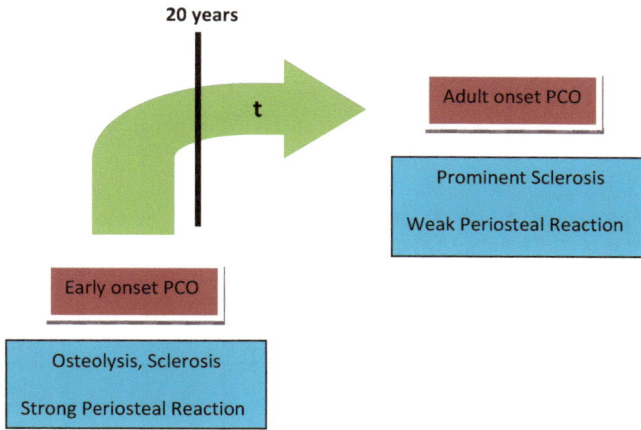

Fig. (6.13). The radiology of Primary Chronic osteomyelitis of the jaws (From Baltensperger 2003, 2004).

Syndrome Associated Primary Chronic Osteomyelitis

a. SAPHO Syndrome

The SAPHO syndrome was first described in **1986 by Chamot and coworkers**.

According to **Kahn and Kahn in 1994** and **Suei *et al.* in 2003**, SAPHO syndrome is a clinical entity combining osteomyelitis, arthritis and skin disease including palmoplantar pustulosis, pustular psoriasis or severe acne [72].

According to **Kahn in 1994**, it is a chronic disorder which involves the skin, bones, and joints. SAPHO is an acronym that stands for morbid alteration of the dermatoskeletal system: synovitis; acne; pustulosis; hyperostosis; and osteitis. The clinical picture is determined by chronic inflammation of one tissue or a combination of any of these tissues [70].

According to Kahn *et al.* in 1994, There are Three Diagnostic Criteria which Can Characterize SAPHO Syndrome [70]

1. Multifocal osteomyelitis with or without skin manifestations
2. Sterile acute or chronic joint inflammation associated with either pustular psoriasis or palmoplantar pustulosis, acne, or hidradenitis
3. Sterile osteitis in the presence of one of the skin manifestations

According to **Kahn and Kahn in 1994**, presence of one of the above mentioned three criteria is sufficient to establish the diagnosis SAPHO syndrome. However, it is still difficult to achieve a definite diagnosis. Clinical (Table **7**), radiological, and histopathological data must also be taken into account for this reason.

In the past two decades many authors like **Kahn** *et al.* **in 1994, Suei** *et al.* **in 1996, Schilling** *et al.* **in 1999; Eyrich** *et al.* **in 1999,** and **Fleuridas** *et al.* **in 2002** have described a possible relationship between SAPHO syndrome and primary chronic osteomyelitis of the jaws [8].

Table 7. Main clinical pictures of SAPHO syndrome which must be seen as a nosological heterogeneous group are summarized in Table below. (Adapted from Schilling 2004).

S.No	Clinical picture of SAPHO syndrome
1.	Chronic recurrent multifocal osteomyelitis in children and adolescent
2.	Chronic recurrent multifocal osteomyelitis in adults
3.	Inflammatory anterior thoracic wall syndrome
4.	Acne + chronic recurrent multifocal osteomyelitis
5.	Triad: chronic recurrent multifocal osteomyelitis + Crohn's disease + palmo-plantar pustulosis
6.	Recurrent multifocal periostitis
7.	Pustulo-psoriatic hyperostotic spondylarthritis
8.	Sterno-costo-clavicular hyperostosis
9.	Acne + spondylarthritis
10.	Primary chronic osteomyelitis of the jaw

Kahn *et al.* **in 1994** and **Suei** *et al.* **in 1996** offered evidence that primary chronic osteomyelitis (described as DSO in their articles) was the mandibular localization of SAPHO syndrome [70]. In fact, primary chronic osteomyelitis of the jaws with extramandibular involvement and skin lesion had already been described before the term SAPHO syndrome was popularized by **Farnam** *et al.* **in 1984**.

In some instances dermatoskeletal symptoms were preceded by PCO of the jaws while on the contrary, in certain other cases PCO of the jaws was seen to follow the dermatoskeletal symptoms. Henceforth **Baltensperger in 2003**, highlighted and discussed the importance of detailed history and thorough clinical examination of the patients presenting with PCO of the jaws in order not to miss the symptoms indicating a possible SAPHO syndrome in the same [8]. Radiographically, the mandibular lesion of the disease present with characteristic findings [72]. The findings include the mixed pattern, solid-type periosteal reaction, external bone resorption, and bone enlargement [72].

Suei *et al.* **in 2003** advocated that the periosteum is a possible site of the original osteomyelitic lesion in SAPHO syndrome [72]. Henceforth, bone scans can prove to be a very helpful diagnostic modality so as to detect extragnathic skeletal involvement in such cases. It is considered important because in many cases the extraskeletal involvement is with clinically silent behavior. On the contrary, according to **Kahn in 1994**, it is also mandatory to rule out involvement of the jaws in cases diagnosed with SAPHO syndrome [8,70]. The involvement of the sternoclavicular joint and palmoplantar pustulosis were the most frequent extragnathic symptoms found. Although **Baltensperger in 2003** mentioned that some of the radiological differences are age related in this disease, however no specific radiological features were observed in the syndrome-associated cases as compared with cases from the same age group with no further dermatoskeletal involvement [8].

According to **Suei *et al.* in 2003**, corticosteroids were found to be more effective than antibiotics in reducing the symptoms due to SAPHO syndrome. Hence, on the basis of the above fact, inspite of considering bacterial etiology for the disease, **Kahn & Kahn in 1994** and **Suei *et al.* in 2003** suggested the main cause for SAPHO syndrome to be an allergic or an autoimmune disorder [72].

b. Chronic Recurrent Multifocal Osteomyelitis

According to **Otsuka and Kayahara in 1999**, Chronic Recurrent Multifocal Osteomyelitis (CRMO) is an inflammatory bone disease resembling infectious osteomyelitis, but showing no obvious infectious origin [73]. Since its first description by **Giedion *et al.* in 1972**, more than 100 cases have been documented in children and adolescents [73].

The term Chronic Recurrent Multifocal Osteomyelitis (CRMO) was first used by **Bjorkstenet *et al.* in 1978** [74]. The clinical features of the affected bone are similar to those in diffuse Sclerosing Osteomyelitis. It is a rare inflammatory bone disease, which affects one or more bones with periods of exacerbation and remission and generally without any infectious agents being isolated from affected areas. Systemic involvement is exceptional and associated cutaneous lesions are common, particularly pustulosis palmoplantaris.

According to **Suei *et al.* in 1994**, the most often affected bones are sternum, clavicle, ribs, spine, pelvis and peripheral long bones including the jaws [75].

According to **Otsuka *et al.* in 1999**, CRMO is a relapsing inflammatory disorder involving multiple bones, most commonly the metaphysis of the long bones [73,89]. **Benedetta *et al.* in 1978** advocated that isolated involvement of the mandible is rare and multiple lesions may occur. According to **Otsuka *et al.* in 1999**, only three cases of CRMO involving the mandible have been reported till then [73].

Epidemiology

Chronic Recurrent Multifocal Osteomyelitis is considered to be an extremely rare disease with no concrete epidemiological data on incidence or prevalence published so far. However, according to **Girschick in 1998 and 2002**, the incidence might be around 1:1,000,000.

Suei *et al.* in 1994 admitted that the disease was predominant in children, but cases in adults have also been noted which seem to be significantly less frequent [75]. He also found the disease to be more common in females than males [75]. **Schilling and coworkers in 2000** noted that with advancing age, there is an increased incidence of palmoplantar pustulosis (a part of SAPHO syndrome) in such patients.

According to **Chamot *et al.* in 1994** and **Schilling and Kessler in 1998**, CRMO has been integrated into nosological heterogenous SAPHO syndrome because of its possible relationship with other dermatoskeletal-associated diseases [8].

Etiology

According to **Flygare *et al.* in 1997**, it represents a distinct clinical entity of unknown cause associated with a confounding and obtuse differential diagnosis [74]. **Suei *et al.* in 1994** considered low grade infection to be sometimes associated with CRMO, but the bacterial cultures were negative in all those reported cases [75].

Clinical Features

According to **Otsuka *et al.* in 1999**, the clinical course of CRMO is unpredictable, with repeated exacerbations and remissions. However according to **Cyrlak in 1986**, it has a self- limited course, with spontaneous remission within several months to 15 years [73].

Suei *et al.* in 1994 and **1995** stressed upon the fact that CRMO is an uncommon disease that is characterized clinically and radiologically by multiple osteomyelitic bone lesions [75,76]. According to **Suei *et al.* in 1994**, patients with CRMO present with an insidious onset involving pain and swelling of the affected area, restricted to one or more bones [75]. Systemic manifestations including fever and weight loss habitually occur during the acute phase of the disease.

According to **Cyrlak and Paris in 1986**, the course of the disease often continues for more than several years [75,77]. Chronic recurrent multifocal osteomyelitis within the pediatric age group can be associated with a number of cutaneous manifestations like pustulosis palmoplantaris (considered by some dermatologists to be a variant of psoriasis vulgaris), diffuse pustulosis, psoriasis vulgaris, acne, Sweet's syndrome and pyoderma gangrenosum [75].

According to **Suei** *et al.* **in 1994**, CRMO is a rare condition that occurs in more than two bones in the body [75].

Radiographic Features

Radiographic findings are similar to septic osteomyelitis, with osteolytic lesions and circumscribed sclerosis.

According to **Suei** *et al.* and **Krutchkoff & Runstad in 1989**, radiography shows osteolytic destruction and periosteal changes to be more apparent in the early stage of the disease, followed by progressive sclerosis in the chronic stage [74]. A similar characterization of CRMO was made by **Cyrlak and Paris** in the long bones [74]. **Mortensson in 1988** and **Suei** *et al.* **in 1994** revealed that Scintigraphy is useful for detecting asymptomatic or silent lesions, showing an increase in deposition in the affected areas [75,78]. Nuclear magnetic resonance or computerized tomography is not essential for diagnosis but is useful to show the extent of lesions and the involvement of joints and adjacent soft tissues.

Diagnosis

Clinical diagnosis is often challenging owing to significant variability in the the clinical picture and course of the disease. **Suei** *et al.* **in 1994** in his review concluded that DSO is an expression of CRMO [74].

Histological analysis of the bony lesions of patients presenting with CRMO patients may prove to be beneficial so as to differentiate them from other bone pathologies especially malignancy [8]. However, the findings may then even resemble acute and secondary chronic osteomyelitis caused by microbiological infection. Therefore, **Girschick in 2002** advocated towards extensive microbiological work-up of the tissue biopsy, including Polymerase Chain Reaction technique. It was considered important so as to establish the diagnosis which will further help to decide on the treatment plan.

It is evident from the discussion above that bone biopsy is considered important so as to arrive at a pertinent diagnosis. Henceforth proper care and caution must be practiced to avoid contamination of the biopsy sample during the time when the sample is harvested from the lesion in question. While lesions of CRMO in the mandible may be easier to access, an oral approach hence should be avoided. A biopsy from another part of the skeleton may therefore be of more diagnostic value, despite a possibly more invasive procedure to harvest the specimen.

Biopsies do not generally find evidence of infectious agents. Biopsies show that lesions are not septic and that this agent functions as a trigger for the immunological and inflammatory reactions. Histopathological investigation of the bone lesions returns variable results.

According to **Bjorksten in 1980**, the initial lesion is characterized by the presence of neutrophils, and is classed as a pseudo- abscess [75,76]. **Suei *et al.* in 1994** also confirmed these findings. He further stated that the chronic lesion has a predominance of lymphocytes with the occasional presence of plasmacytes, histiocytes and fibrosis [75 - 79].

Various Authors Have Suggested Different Diagnostic Criteria for CRMO Which are as Follows:

King *et al.* in 1987 suggested the following criteria

  i. Multifocal bony lesions which are diagnosed clinically or radiographically.
 ii. Prolonged course of the disease over 6 months duration which is marked by varying activity of disease and with most patients being healthy between recurrent episodes of pain, swelling and tenderness.
iii. Lack of response to antimicrobial therapy given for at least 1 month.

Manson *et al.* in 1989 proposed the following Diagnostic criteria for CRMO [75]

  i. Evidence of two or more than two radiographically confirmed bony lesions
 ii. Evidence of a prolonged course of at least six months with characteristic exacerbations and remission
iii. Evidence of Osteomyelitic changes radiographically and with nuclear scintigraphy
iv. Evidence of no response towards antimicrobial therapy for at least one month
 v. Lack of identifiable cause

Recent studies suggest the following criteria for a diagnosis of CRMO

• Duration of more than three months [93]
• Histological evidence of chronic bone inflammation, excluding other diseases
• An absence of bacterial growth in cultures.

According to **Suei *et al.* in 1994**, test results reveal elevated Erythrocytic Sedimentation Rate [75] and C- Reactive Protein during the acute phase which normalizes during remissions. Cultures are habitually negative for bacteria, fungi and mycobacteria. However, Propionibacterium acnes in bone aspirate may be associated with CMRO.

CHAPTER 7

Osteomyelitis of Jaws *vs.* Long Bones

Abstract: As it has been already discussed, osteomyelitis can be defined as the inflammation in the medullary portion of the bone. But this does not mean that the osteomyelitis of the jaws will be similar to that of long bones. According to several authors there exists a difference in the pathogenesis of osteomyelitis of long bones when compared with the jaws. This is considered important because the management of a particular disease depends upon the pathogenesis. Since the pathogenesis of osteomyelitis of jaws is considered different by certain authors as compared to the osteomyelitis of long bones, the treatment protocol of both these entities cannot be similar. This particular chapter will highlight the difference in the pathogenesis of osteomyeliis of long bones and the jaws.

Keywords: Comparison of osteomyelitis of jaws and long bones, Osteomyelitis of jaws, Osteomyelitis of Long bones, Pathogenesis of osteomyelitis of jaws.

According to **Donohue and Abelardo in 1970**, there exists difference of opinion in pathogenesis of osteomyelitis when seen in the long bones and in the jaws [80].

Hence before discussing the management of osteomyelitis of the jaws, it seems pretty important to understand the differences between osteomyelitis of the long bones and the jaws.

Some authors like **Turek in 1959** and **Thoma in 1960**, advocated the removal of teeth in the presence of acute infection, while in contrast several others like **Bailey in 1956** and **Davis in 1960** have cautioned against the removal of a tooth with an acute alveolar abscess [80].

According to **Turek in 1959**, in the long bones, the most frequent cause of infection is septicaemia in the younger age groups. The next most common cause occurs as a complication of fractures and is more common in adults.

In contrast, according to **Warren in 1963**, osteomyelitis of the jaws is rarely due to hematogenous spread. The great majority of cases involving the jaws are due to complications of a primary dental infection while a lesser number arise as a complication of a fracture of the bone.

Deepak Gupta, Soheyl Skeikh & Shambulingappa Pallagatti

According to **Donohue and Abelardo in 1970,** in both cases the source of the infection is external [80]. The causative organism in osteomyelitis of the limb bones is usually a hemolytic staphylococcus, with streptococci being somewhat less frequently responsible. In the jaws, however, because the infection arises as a complication of dental caries, we are dealing with a mixed infection where the haemolytic streptococcus is frequently the predominant organism.

According to **Donohue and Abelardo in 1970,** the evolution of the disease in the two regions varies. In the long bones, the infection arrives at the metaphysis *via* the blood stream if it is due to a hematogenous infection, and involves the diaphysis later. On occasion, the infection is introduced from the exterior as a complication of trauma. In either circumstance the resultant osteomyelitis develops in a bone with a relatively thick cortex.

In the jaws, the conditions are different. As already mentioned, the infection is most often introduced from the exterior, usually owing to dental caries but occasionally through a fracture site [80].

The maxilla is composed almost entirely of spongy bone with a very thin cortex. Any infectious process of this bone can either remain localized or can spread into the soft tissues resulting in a cellulitis, fistula or sinusitis. According to **Fullmer** *et al.* **in 2006**, osteomyelitis of the maxilla is rare [81] because of its anatomical structure.

According to **Donohue and Abelardo in 1970,** in the jaws, the bone is separated from the mouth by the relatively thin oral mucosa. Hence an infective process arising from a tooth may easily erode the thin alveolar cortical bone and secondarily involve the soft tissues. If, however, as occasionally happens in the mandible, the roots of the tooth are midway between the lateral and medial cortical plates and if the roots are sufficiently long, or if the vertical height of the body or alveolar process of the mandible is short, then the apex of the tooth will be in the central region of the mandibular bone marrow, surrounded by a relatively thick layer of cortical bone. Infections arising from such teeth might develop as osteomyelitis.

Depending on the clinical course of the disease, the surgical treatment of osteomyelitis of the long bones consists of antibiotic therapy, early drainage and later sequestrectomy and saucerization. These techniques alone, however, are not adequate in treating this disease of the jaws, as illustrated by the cases presented by **Donohue and Abelardo in 1970.** In the mandible and maxilla there is the added factor of the presence of teeth.

According to **Calhoun** *et al.* **in 1988**, it is essential that the teeth involved in the infection be treated at the outset of the disease so as not to prolong the condition unnecessarily and mutilate the patient [82].

Other Points in Treatment Deserve Emphasis

Firstly, according to **Calhoun** *et al.* **in 1988,** the reason for removing infected teeth in the case of an acute dentoalveolar abscess is to eliminate the cause of the disease and establish drainage [82].

According to **Donohue and Abelardo in 1970,** these objectives can frequently be attained by antibiotic therapy, endodontia and apical curettage without removing the tooth [80].

Secondly, some authors have advocated the use of hot, moist compresses in the treatment of osteomyelitis of the jaws. **Donohue and Abelardo in 1970,** however, contend that the use of heat in bone infections serves to spread rather than contain the infection.

Thirdly, according to **Calhoun** *et al.* **in 1988,** in cases of osteomyelitis of the jaws, decortication, sequestrectomy and saucerization can frequently be carried out [82] by an intraoral approach, thus avoiding disfiguring scars. When indicated, immediate reconstruction, using a free bone graft to the mandible can also be carried out by the oral route.

CHAPTER 8

MANAGEMENT – General Considerations

Abstract: The management of osteomyelitis was an issue of great debate and research since long. The treatment of osteomyelitis has been practiced by various clinicians. Literature also reveals that the treatment of osteomyelitis of jaws was practiced since the year1900. There are three treatment protocols advocated for osteomyelitis which vary from simple non-invasive approach like antimicrobial therapy to more invasive and radical treatment like surgical removal of the affected part. The nonsurgical approach includes various medicinal treatment options including antibiotics,anti-inflammatory and muscle relaxants. There is evidence of certain other conservative non surgical management approaches like hyperbaric oxygen therapy and bisphosphonate treatment too. If the dental professional considers that the non surgical approach may not fetch required results; then a surgical intervention is considered. This may include decortications alone or with bone grafting and partial or segmental resection. Unfortunately, there still exist dilemmas as to what approach to be followed in certain cases of osteomyelitis of jaws. This is because of the evidence of multiple recurrences of the disease. Further it is also reported that sometimes aggressive management may lead to significant co-morbidity with subsequent need for reconstructive surgery. Literature also reveals that symptomatic treatment may also be necessary in some cases. Such symptomatic treatment may include debridement of necrotic tissues and foreign materials along with skin closure of unhealed wounds. This present chapter highlights the various treatment protocols instituted and adopted by various researchers worldwide with recommendations for better treatment protocol for the dental professionals.

Keywords: Acute Osteomyelitis, Antimicrobial therapy, Anti-inflammatory, Bisphosphonate therapy, Chronic osteomyelitis, Conservative management of Osteomyelitis of jaws, Decortication, Diabetes Mellitus, Hyperbaric Oxygen therapy, Infantile Osteomyelitis, Management of Osteomyelitis of jaws, Osteochemonecrosis, Osteonecrosis, Osteopetrosis, Primary chronic osteomyelitis, Secondary chronic osteomyelitis, Segmental resection, Surgical management of osteomyelitis of jaws, SAPHO syndrome.

Osteomyelitis was a frequent infection happening to the soldiers injured during the war. It was during the world war when **Baer WS** of Johns Hopkins University in **1931** found that the wounds which were cared for, often suppurated extensively

Deepak Gupta, Soheyl Skeikh & Shambulingappa Pallagatti

while totally neglected but fly-blown cases in which maggots had hatched, healed in a short time with a minimum of disability [83 - 85].

Bear in 1931 further suggested that maggots destroyed the invading bacteria and at the same time removed the devitalized tissue without injuring the healthy portions of the wound. He further proved the effectiveness of maggots by extensive successful experiments. Maggots were then cultured and supplied by various pharmaceutical companies at that time [83].

Livingstone and Prince in 1932 reported the extraction of a bactericidal substance from the crushed maggots. They further used it with and without maggots in a number of cases of human osteomyelitis and observed good results [83 - 86].They also stated that the extract from maggots had the advantage of being relatively sterile and of neither growing nor crawling in the wound [83, 86].

According to **Stewart in 1934**, maggots have large quantities of calcium carbonate in their bodies which is exuded through their wall. This calcium ion is well known to stimulate phagocytosis [83]. **Stewart in 1934** further stated that the calcium carbonate secreted by maggots aid in the natural body defences and could perhaps be substituted for the maggots themselves in the treatment of osteomyelitis [83].

Stewart in 1934 formulated a compound for treatment of osteomyelitis. It consisted of:

  i. **Calcium carbonate** for phagocytic action.
 ii. **Picric acid in dilute solution**. Picric acid was used to stimulate phagocytosis. In addition, it prevented the bacterial leucocoidin from destroying the phagocytes. This leucocoidin was secreted by the infecting bacteria in the wound. It is a white cell destroyer and kills phagocytes as soon as it comes in contact with them.
iii. **Glycerin** to reduce the surface tension. Glycerine was added to picric acid in small amounts to enhance the penetration of picric acid in the crevices of the wounds.

Stewart in 1934 experimented laboratory animals and good results were obtained. Subsequently 41 human subjects were treated by this method. In human cases according to **Stewart in 1934**, necrotic bone was first removed surgically and then the wound was packed for 24 hours. Then it was irrigated with picric acid glycerine solution. Shortly after this, the aqueous calcium carbonate suspension was sprayed into the wound.

According to **Bear in 1934,** the calcium picrate formed in the wound has analgesic properties beneficial to the patient [8].

According to **Mckeever in 2008**, while the beneficial effects of maggots in wounds particularly in osteomyelitis have been documented over the years, still they have never gained widespread use. Nonetheless, the United States Food and Drug Administration approved the use of sterile maggots in 2004 [84].

According to **Adekeye** *et al.* **in 1985**, the treatment of osteomyelitis is quite well emphasized in the literature [9].

The goals of management are as follows:

  i. Attenuate and eradicate proliferating pathological organisms
 ii. Promote healing and
iii. Re- establish vascular permeability [16].

As discussed earlier, debridement of infected and necrotic tissue is required for the treatment of osteomyelitis of the jaws in order to reduce the bacterial concentration as much as possible. This will allow the body to overcome the infection.

The management includes [16]:

A. Conservative treatment (antibiotics), and
B. Surgical treatment.

Adekeye *et al.* **in 1985** postulated that general management of osteomyelitis must incorporate the treatment of malnutrition along with treatment of any associated debilitating disease [9]. The basic aim is to restore adequate vascularity. **Fang and Galino in 2009** stated that the healing process in osteomyelitis can be fastened with improved local vascularization [87]. This can be achieved with the help of surgical decortications which along with removal and debridement of poorly vascularized tissue, can also bring well-vascularized tissue to the affected bone [8, 87]. This allows antibiotics to reach the target area thus facilitating the healing process [87].

Various researchers have also advocated the usage of Hyperbaric Oxygen therapy in the treatment of the patients with osteomyelitis.

Lantrode *et al.* **in 2007** considered hyperbaric oxygen (HBO) therapy as an established treatment modality for treatment as well as prevention of osteoradionecrosis. However, on the contrary, **Fang and Galino in 2009** revealed that there is no concrete evidence regarding the therapeutic value of HBO therapy in the treatment of Osteomyelitis of jaws [8, 87, 88].

Principles of Therapy Of Acute And Secondary Chronic Osteomyelitis

There has been wide variety of views regarding the principles of treatment of Acute and Secondary chronic osteomyelitis. **Baltenspenger in 2003** highlighted that Acute and Secondary chronic osteomyelitis share similar treatment goals (Table **8**). However certain authors are of the view that the management protocol for acute and secondary chronic osteomyelitis may differ [8]. This was explained on the basis of more prominent pain and discomfort in acute cases (**Leroy in 1986**) as compared to secondary chronic variety. Further secondary chronic osteomyelitis is considered to be more advanced as compared to acute variety because of the difference in time frame for the establishment of bone infection.

Table 8. Therapeutic goals in treatment of acute and secondary chronic osteomyelitis of the jaws *(Adapted from Baltensperger MM, Eyrich GK (eds). Osteomyelitis of jaws, 2009) [8].*

1.	Eradication of infection and removal of infectious focus
2.	Pain management
3.	Limitation of further spreading of the disease
4.	Fracture prophylaxis, and stabilization of infected fractures
5.	Preservation of anatomic structures when possible
6.	Prevention of relapse of disease
7.	Prevention of chronification of the infection
8.	Reestablishment of anatomy and function

ACUTE OSTEOMYELITIS

Table 9. Principles of treatment of acute osteomyelitis of the jaws [8].

1.	Establish correct diagnosis, based on history, clinical evaluation, and imaging studies
2.	Biopsy in unclear cases to rule out other pathology (*e.g.*, malignancy)
3.	Determine extent of infected bone and soft tissue
4.	Evaluation and correction of host defence deficiencies when possible prior to surgical intervention
5.	Removal of source of infection, usually a dental focus, foreign bodies/implants, Local incision and drainage of pus, Local curettage with removal of superficial sequestra and saucerization if necessary
6.	Collection of specimens for Gram stain, aerobic and anaerobic culture and sensitivity during the above initial procedures; histopathology
7.	Begin with empiric broad-spectrum antibiotic therapy and change to culture-guided antibiotics as soon as possible
8.	More extensive surgical debridement if necessary (*e.g.*, decortication, resection)
9.	Possible adjunctive hyperbaric oxygen therapy

Correct diagnostic approach and establishment of a correct diagnosis is mandatory for successful treatment of any ailment with better prognosis. Infective processes in acute osteomyelitis leads to vascular insufficiency in the early course of the disease (**Caldwell in 1909 and Bitting in 1929**) [55, 56]. This mandates medical management in the form of appropriate antibiotics in the cases acute osteomyelitis. The antibiotics must be instituted within the first three days after the onset of the symptoms.

According to **Mercuri in 1991**, early detection of the disease is important. This can be done from the patient's history and medical exams.

According to **Walker in 1947**, initiation of early and adequate antibiotic therapy may lead to spontaneous resolution of the disease [9]. But according to **Bitting in 1929**, if the diagnosis and subsequently the treatment are delayed, it may lead to rupture of the periosteum leading to swelling and abscess formation thus necessitating the role of incision and drainage of pus beneath the periosteum [55].

According to **Walker in 1947**, crystalline penicillin, ampicillin, procaine penicillin, streptomycin, lincomycin, clindamycin and metronidazole were the antibiotics administered in osteomyelitis.

Adekeye *et al.* **in 1985** found metronidazole to be very effective when used in combination with the above mentioned antibiotics as it is effective against anaerobes [9]. The value of metronidazole alone in the treatment of dental sepsis has been shown by **Ingham** *et al.* **in 1977** [9].

The potency of metronidazole in the resolution of dry socket was demonstrated by **Rood and Murgatroyd in 1979** [9]. It was called as localized osteomyelitis by **Israel in 1976**.

According to **Alabadi and Nikpoor in 1994**, radiological imaging ranging from conventional radiology to advance is mandatory for the confirmation of the suspected diagnosis as well as to delineate the lesion extent [26]. Advanced radiological approach may include CT scan and/or MRI scan. However if these diagnostic modalities are not of sufficient diagnostic value, in such cases Radionuclide scans may be deemed necessary. Radionuclide scans are capable of tracing the infection at an even early stage when the CT or MRI fails to provide any clue in the suspected lesion [26].

As discussed earlier, removal of the causative factor is mandatory for healing process to initiate [8]. Such removal of the causative agent leads to decompression of the acute intramedullary as well as subperiosteal regions of the bone affected with osteomyelitis of the jaws. This decompression is required so as to resolve subsequent vascular and cortical compression thus resolving the progression of the disease [8]. Further, there must be early recognition and addressal of the factors which can lead to reduced local tissue perfusion as this will strongly influence the therapy and treatment outcome.

According to **Bitting in 1929**, the dominant factor in the treatment is the relief of tension beneath the periosteum [55] and in the cancellous bone. According to **Oechsner in 1914**, this release of tension is accomplished by making an incision over the point of greatest tenderness through the soft tissues and periosteum to the bone [59].

Archer in 1975 advocated early hospitalization and administration of massive doses of penicillin with adequate fluid and dietary intake. He also emphasized upon the importance of rest in such cases [9].

Mercuri in 1991 emphasized consultation of appropriate medical specialist so as to resolve many of these underlying problems [8].

Important clues can be achieved regarding the initial diagnosis by the quality of pus as shown in Table **10**. Pus can be collected with the help of sterile, large-gauge needles and the pus and other material removed by debridement should be transported under anaerobic conditions. **Baltensperger and Eyrich in 2000** advocated the practice of correct mucosal and skin preparation for specimen collection [8]. Gram stains may be helpful to determine initial antibiotic therapy until laboratory results are available [8].

Table 10. Important clues to initial diagnosis and treatment by the consistency, colour, and odour of pus [8]. *(According to Baltensperger and Eyrich in 2000).*

S.No.	Features of Pus	Clues
1.	Thick creamy pus from a localized abscess	Staphylococcal infection
2.	A foul-smelling, dark exudate accompanying slough of necrotic tissues	Anaerobic osteomyelitis
3.	Gas in soft tissues	Anaerobic osteomyelitis
4.	Multiple organisms in Gram stain of variable morphological characteristics	Anaerobic osteomyelitis

Topazian in 2002 also supported the fact that anaerobic osteomyelitis is suspected on the basis of variable morphology of multiple organisms in Gram stain. He further stated that possible contamination of the specimen collected must be kept in consideration so as to achieve fair microbiological result.

According to **Baltensperger in 2003 and Topazian in 2002**, if the infection shows inadequate response towards the regime, there must be a provision for adjustments in the same [8]. In other words, in such cases repeated cultures must be practiced to ensure correct antibiotic therapy. Further, extensive surgical treatment like decortications and/or resection along with adjunctive HBO therapy can also be considered [8].

Treatment of Infantile Osteomyelitis [16]

The treatment should be prompt and aggressive.

1. **Antibiotics** are preferably given by intravenous route. Penicillins or penicillinase resistant penicillins like flucloxacillin, or broad spectrum antibiotics may be given for 2-4 weeks.
   According to **Jacobi and Sagorin in 1945,** Penicillin therapy revolutionized the prognosis in osteomyelitis of the jaws in infancy. They further stated that, when dealing with such infections, it is not only the threat to life which is considered, but the cosmetic result is also of paramount importance in those who survive [89].
2. **Culture and sensitivity testing**: Culture is taken from the discharge from the sinus tracts and sensitivity testing should be done. The antibiotic regimen is to be modified accordingly.
   Many cases of acute osteomyelitis are cured by antibiotics only. **Schenk in 1948** reported five cases of infantile osteomyelitis treated with penicillin. All of his patients were cured without loss of tooth germs.
3. **Incision and drainage of fluctuant areas**: It is indicated in the presence of periosteal or palatal abscesses.
   This procedure was followed by **Goldbloom and Bacal** in his patients in **1937 [90]**.
4. **Irrigations**: In case of sinus tracts, irrigations are done frequently.
5. **Supportive therapy**:
   i. Analgesics such as Ibuprofen 400 – 600 mg thrice daily, anti-inflammatory agents such as Ibuprofen 400 mg and antipyretic agents such as Paracetamol 500 mg thrice daily.
   ii. Fluids
   iii. Proper diet.
   Proteins and multivitamins such as niacinamide 50 mg, L- glutamic acid 100 mg, vitamin B_2 1.5 mg and d-panthenol 50 mg should be supplied abundantly.
6. **Sequestrectomy or removal of necrotic tooth germs**: Removal of sequestra is on the basis of clinical and radiological findings when there is evidence of complete separation of the sequestra from the surrounding bone.

According to Golgbloom and Bacal in 1937, surgical interference should be conservative as loss of bone and teeth leads to severe deformities in the later life

[90].

According to **Jacobi and Sagorin in 1945**, loss of tooth buds in infants may lead to deformity and disfigurement when the teeth erupt later on [89].

Jacobi and Sagorin in 1945 further stated that loss of tooth buds in the upper jaw is not likely to result in deformity, but when tooth buds are lost from the lower jaw, the loss is more serious as the shape of the upper dental arch appears to be controlled by the shape of the lower arch [89].

Hence,**Jacobi and Sagorin in 1945** concluded that since the loss of tooth buds is partly due to surgical intervention, it is obvious that the usage of penicillin will lead to minimal surgery and hence minimum deformity due to loss of primary dentition [89].

According to **Dunphy and Frazer in 1945,** children, who have undergone sequestrectomies, should be followed up by an orthodontist to aid in the development of the arch and maintenance of occlusion [91].

According to **Dunphy and Frazer in 1945**, intramuscular and local penicillin and sulfadiazine can adequately handle the infectious process in acute osteomyelitis of the maxilla in infants. Bone sequestration, prolonged drainage, and facial deformity can hence be prevented [91].

According to **Wilensky in 1932**, abscesses in association with the lower jaw in infantile osteomyelitis are simpler technically and ordinary surgical principles should be followed in treating them. He further stated that sequestra should not be removed until involucrum formation is abundant [92, 93].

SECONDARY CHRONIC OSTEOMYELITIS

As stated previously, the principles of therapy and management of secondary chronic osteomyelitis is similar to the cases of acute osteomyelitis. Since SCO represents infection at a more advanced stage, henceforth radiological imaging is considered to be more conclusive in secondary chronic osteomyelitis as compared to the cases of acute nature [94].

As a part of management of pathological fractures in long bones, **Calandruccio in 1971** advocated alignment and immobilization in addition to drainage, antibiotic therapy and sequestrectomy.

Adekeye *et al.* in 1985 suggested the use of this principle in the pathological fractures in case of maxillofacial osteomyelitis as well. CT scans are considered as a gold standard diagnostic imaging modality in the determination of the extent of the lesion prior to surgery.

According to **Johnston** and **Conly in 2007**, the only difference in the principle of management lies in the fact that surgical debridement is a mainstay of management for chronic osteomyelitis [94,95]. On the contrary this is not frequently practiced in the acute form [94].

Further the other surgical treatment modalities like Decortication and resection are considered early in secondary chronic osteomyelitis while in acute cases it is done as a last resort when more extensive surgical debridement is required.

According to **Adekeye** *et al.* **in 1985**, affected bone of the jaws requires resection in case the buccal and medial cortical plates are destructed by the osteomyelitis that too without an evidence of new bone formation [9].

There has been debate regarding the usage of antibiotics in secondary chronic osteomyelitis. According to **Lazzarini** *et al.* **in 2002** and **2005**, both antibiotic and surgical treatment are required in chronic osteomyelitis cases [9]. Surgical debridement is considered to be the initial treatment in SCO. Further antibiotics should only be prescribed based on culture report. However in daily practice, most of the cases of SCO have already been pre-treated with antibiotics without any culture report.

Tissue samples are considered to be more reliable for obtaining cultures as compared to swabs (**Marx 1991**). This was attributed to the fact that swab cultures of pus or putrid exudate often contain mostly dead microorganisms.

According to **Baltensperger in 2003**, high-dose antibiotic therapy is initiated in cases of SCO at frequent intervals after surgical debridement. As in cases of acute osteomyelitis, the initial antibiotic management of secondary chronic osteomyelitis of the jaws is empiric at this stage. However the choice of antibiotic should be based on clinical observations at the time of surgery such as as color, odor and consistency of pus and tissue [8].

In general, according to **LeRoy in 1986**, initial antibiotic regime will consist of a broad-spectrum drug having a bactericidal character with a low toxicity [63]. Adjustments can be made as soon as sufficient culture data is available [63]. Patients with osteomyelitis usually require treatment as in-patients.

Repeated hospitalizations were seldom required, except for complicated cases involving repeated surgical procedures.

According to **Johnston and Conly in 2007**, treatment guidelines for acute and chronic osteomyelitis in adults should include prolonged courses of intravenous antimicrobials [94].

The antibiotic therapy in acute and chronic osteomyelitis should be stopped on the basis of empiric judgement depending upon clinical evaluation as well as follow up imaging features.

According to **Baltensperger and Eyrich in 2000,** this clinical evaluation is based upon the evidence of cessation of suppuration and adequate healing of the surgical wound [8]. There must be complete resolution of the all four cardinal signs of infection which includes rubor, tumor, calor, dolor and impaired function [8]. Imaging should highlight resolution of osteolysis and sequester. It can also reveal some early bone remodelling. In general, antibiotic therapy may therefore be extended for a period of 4–6 weeks after surgery [8].

In cases of persistent infection, adjunctive hyperbaric oxygen therapy as advocated by **LeRoy in 1986** [63] and possibility of further surgical debridement must be evaluated.

Secondary Chronic Osteomyelitis Associated with Bone Pathology and/or Systemic Disease

It is a well known fact that the underlying cause facilitating osteomyelitis has a great impact on the management. Henceforth, the cases of SCO of the jaws associated with any local or systemic disease deserve to be mentioned separately.

Secondary Chronic Osteomyelitis Associated with Bone Pathology

Baltensperger and Eyrich in 2000 [8] highlighted that the host defences are usually impaired in the cases of SCO associated with underlying bony pathology. Henceforth the physiological bone response that includes neo-osteogenesis, periostitis and sequester formation due to osteoblastic and osteoclastic activity may be either less prominent or even absent in such cases [8]. Thus, diagnosis can be challenging. Preferably concomitant pathology facilitating infection is addressed as early as possible in the therapeutic process. In cases of underlying bone pathology this is not possible [8]. Principally, it must be differentiated between a localized and generalized systemic bone pathology. This differentiation has a big impact on the proposed surgical therapy.

a. **Localized bone pathology:**

A typical example for this type of localized bone pathology is infected osteoradionecrosis. According to **Wong *et al.* in 1997,** osteoradionecrosis of the jaws is one of the most serious complications of radiation therapy for head and neck malignancies [97]. Further he also stated that the criteria used to define osteoradionecrosis vary [97].

Marx and Johnson in 1987 have defined osteoradionecrosis as "an exposure of irradiated bone which fails to heal without intervention."

Epstein and Wong in 1987 described osteoradionecrosis as spontaneously healing, slowly progressive, or rapidly progressive and symptomatic [97].

According to **Epstein and Wong in 1987** and **Beumer J** *et al.* **in 1983**, osteoradionecrosis lesions may respond with minimal conservative intervention [97].

Rankow R in 1971 and **Brumer J in 1984** also supported the above fact [97].

In contrast to the above mentioned statement, **Marx R in 1983** and **Morten M in 1986**, advocated that some lesions of osteoradionecrosis respond only to invasive surgery and hyperbaric oxygen therapy [97].

Barak S in 1988 and **Mounsey RA in 1993** also supported this fact [97].

According to **van Merkesteyn** *et al.* **in 1994**, once osteoradionecrosis develops, it may require surgical resection in substantial percentage of the patients [98]. Hence, surgical therapy in such cases may be more extensive. Apart of involving the affected bone, the surgery is even extended to regions of vital bone which are not affected by the infection and the underlying bone pathology.

According to **Marx R in 1983**, conservative approaches have been cited to be wasteful when they prove to be ineffective involving unacceptable amount of time, effort and cost.

According to **Marx in 1985**, when hyperbaric oxygen was used in a high risk population who required tooth removal in irradiated mandibles, incidence of osteoradionecrosis was 5.4% as compared to 29.9% with the antibiotic group [99]. Hence, hyperbaric oxygen therapy should be considered as a prophylactic measure when post-irradiation dental care involving any traumatic procedure is desired to be performed on the patient [99].

Baltensperger in 2003 reported that the effect of antibiotic therapy in such cases is less effective. This is attributed to diminished local vascularisation of the bone post radiation. This hinders the establishment of sufficient concentration of antibiotics in the target area thus reducing their effectivity.

According to **van Merkesteyn** *et al.* **in 1994**, Hyperbaric Oxygen therapy (HBO) may prove as a boon in such cases as this may increase bone vascularisation [98].

Henceforth HBO therapy may help to limit resection [98].

b. Bone Pathology of Systemic Nature:

According to **Baltensperger and Eyrich in 2000**, a different treatment approach is required in the cases with underlying bone pathology of systemic nature [8]. This is so because potentially all the bones of the body may be affected by this condition.

A typical representative of this group is

i. Osteonecrosis or Osteochemonecrosis
ii. Osteopetrosis (Albers–Schonberg disease)

Osteonecrosis or Osteochemonecrosis

This condition, also described as bis-phossy jaw, has become strikingly more prominent in recent years.

According to **Hewitt and Farah in 2007**, it is caused by bisphosphonate therapy [100]. According to **Baltensperger and Eyrich in 2000**, chemotherapeutic medications can predispose to osteochemonecrosis of the jaw. However, bisphosphonates are known to be most commonly associated with Osteochemonecrosis of the jaws [8].

According to **Pires *et al.* in 2005**, concomitant intake of steroids can contribute to development of osteonecrosis as corticosteroids demonstrate antiangiogenic and immunosuppressive properties [101].

Further, according to **Koo *et al.* in 2002**, the threshold needed to induce osteonecrosis due to steroid consumption has been estimated to be 1800 mg/month [101].

Brooks JK *et al.* in 2007 also agreed to the above mentioned fact.

According to **Hewitt and Farah in 2007**, Bisphosphonates appear to express their effects at cell, tissue and molecular level. He further reviewed that the pathogenesis of Bisphosphonate related osteonecrosis centres on Bisphosphonate induced osteoclast inhibition or secondarily in terms of antiangiogenic mechanisms [100].

According to **Ruggiero in 2004** and **Chiandussi in 2006**, Bisphosphonates act through the inhibition of bone resorption by reducing osteoclastic activity [102, 103].

This alteration limits the ability of bone healing after trauma and therefore makes the bone tissue more susceptible to secondary bacterial infection.

According to **Brooks JK in 2007**, surgical intervention is accompanied by a high complication rate in osteonecrosis because of the reduced healing capacity of bone [101]. Therefore, according to **Baltensperger and Eyrich in 2000**, in cases of osteochemonecrosis of the jaw complicated by osteomyelitis, surgery should be limited to a minimal debridement of the necrotic bone and primary closure of the surgical site with a mucoperiosteal flap. Extended antibiotic therapy and possibly hyperbaric oxygen therapy should always be considered as adjunctive treatment modalities [8]. Hence, according to **Ruggiero *et al.* in 2006**, dental examination is required before administering bisphosphonate to the patients.

Hewitt & Farah in 2007 and **Brooks JK *et al.* in 2007** were also with the opinion that a thorough dental examination is required in the patients who are supposed to be treated with intravenous bisphosphonates.

Further authors like **Ruggerio *et al.* in 2006** revealed that the procedures which involve bone healing must be completed before the initiation of bisphosphonate therapy whenever possible. The patients must also be intimated for maintaining good oral hygiene and for frequent dental follow up visits.

Osteopetrosis

Osteoperrosis is another systemic disease or condition which affects the bone and the jaws. According to **Ahmed I *et al.* in 2006**, it is also known as Albers–Schonberg disease or marble bone disease [104].

Ögütcen-Toller *et al.* in 2010 mentioned osteopetrosis as a genetically inherited disease. The bones of the patients presenting with this disease progressively become less vascular with increased mineral content [105].

According to **Lawoyin DO *et al.* in 1987**, patients with osteopetrosis seem to be especially susceptible to osteomyelitis [2, 10, 104]. **Ahmed I *et al.*** also concluded the above mentioned fact in 2006.

Osteopetrosis affects the bone by progressive reduction in perfusion. It also leads to reduced cellular content of the bone along with. Furthermore, there is gradual ossification of the medullar component of the bone. This leads to reduced functioning of the marrow further resulting in anemia and leukopenia [8, 10, 104]. In accordance with other systemic pathologies affecting bone as the main target tissue as discussed above in this chapter, osteopetrosis when complicated by secondary chronic osteomyelitis of the jaws can be best managed by minimal surgical intervention whenever possible [8, 10, 104]. This is attributed to hypovascular and hypocellular bone in these patients resulting in limited healing capacity.

According to **Ahmed I *et al.* in 2006**, medical management of osteomyelitis in a patient suffering from osteopetrosis is also based upon the efforts to stimulate host osteoclasts [104].

Secondary Chronic Osteomyelitis associated with Systemic Disease

As mentioned above, systemic conditions which can facilitate the development and progress of acute and secondary chronic osteomyelitis of the jaws must be addressed as early as possible in the treatment cascade.

These include:

i. **Diabetes:**
According to **Chukwudum U *et al.* in 2009**, diabetes can influence the development and continuation of osteomyelitis [106].
Leukocytes of diabetic patients have a reduced life span. Further they also represent diminished chemotaxis as well as phagocytosis. In addition to this, diabetes lead to micro- and macroangiopathy which further reduces tissue perfusion. This results in failure of the individual to mount an effective inflammatory response. The delivery of antibiotics to the target area and wound healing is also diminished.
Henceforth, the treatment of osteomyelitis of the jaws in diabetic patients must include a more aggressive surgical intervention and wound care. In addition to diabetic control, antibiotics and adjunctive therapy such as hyperbaric oxygen therapy is also required.

ii. **Leukemia:**
According to **Baltensperger in 2000**, Since Leukemia strongly affects the function and number of white blood cells, it can favourably predispose the patient to osteomyelitis of the jaws [8]. Further, treatment of Leukemia by chemotherapy is also known to reduce the general healing capacity [8] in the patient.
Malignant proliferation of white blood cells within the marrow causes crowding of the blood cells. This decreases the formation of red blood cells (RBC's) leading to myelodysplastic anemia. This condition reduces tissue oxygenation and therefore further reduces leukocyte and macrophage microbial killing ability.
According to **Baltensperger and Eyrich in 2000**, empiric broad spectrum antibiotics are prescribed at the start of the treatment of such patients with leukemia and secondary chronic osteomyelitis of the jaws. Further those broad

spectrum antibiotics must be culture guided as soon as possible [8]. The surgical phase of the protocol in these patients should be delayed by approximately 2 weeks after chemotherapy is sustained and functional white blood cells have recovered.

To coordinate appropriate treatment, consultation with an oncologist is necessary [8].

iii. **Anaemia:**

According to **Olaitan AA *et al.* in 1997**, osteomyelitis of the jaws can occur in sickle cell anemia patients [107]. Although, sporadic cases have been reported, it may promote acute and secondary chronic osteomyelitis of the jaws *via* systemic debilitation, reduced tissue oxygenation, and bone infarction.

According to **Marx in 1991,** anaemic children who are homozygous for the anemia trait are especially predisposed to develop osteomyelitis. Usually intensive and aggressive management of the anemia as well as the osteomyelitis is required on an inpatient setting with close cooperation of the involved medical disciplines [8].

According to **Olaitan AA *et al.* in 1997,** Osteomyelitis of the jaws in sickle cell disease has been treated with antibiotics either alone or in combination with surgery [107].

According to **Olaitan AA *et al.* in 1997,** during sickling crises, anaesthesia and surgery are avoided and management is limited to treatment of symptoms and alleviation of pain [107].

iv. **Intravenous Drug Abusers:**

Intravenous drug abusers may develop chronic osteomyelitis through repeated septic injections or by harbouring septic vegetations on heart valves, in the skin, or within veins that produce periodic septic emboli.

v. **Poor Oral Hygiene:**

According to **Baltensperger and Eyrich in 2000**, poor oral hygiene and the concomitant development of dental foci raise the risk for infection. Besides an aggressive medical and surgical approach, nutritional support is advisable. Maintaining compliance in these patients for prolonged antibiotic therapy is a further challenge [8].

vi. **Patients with Significant Immunodeficiency:**

According to **Asseri L *et al.* in 1997**, patients suffering from AIDS seems to develop a higher rate of acute and secondary chronic osteomyelitis of the jaws as compared to a general healthy population [3]. In these patients, osteomyelitis of the jaws progresses faster with less clinical symptoms and is less responsive to conservative/minimal invasive therapy approaches. Therefore, the disease often transforms to a chronic stage.

According to **Marx in 1991,** cultures also frequently reveal unusual organisms in combination with more common oral pathogens. These may include

Candida species most of the times. Sometimes Actinomyces and Nocardial species have also been reported [8].

According to **Asseri L *et al.* in 1997,** the treatment of osteomyelitis of the jaws in AIDS patients is addressed towards sustaining some comfort [107]. Further the treatment should be aggressive surgically and medically. Antibiotics should be culture oriented as soon as possible. Concomitant treatment of opportunistic infections and antiviral therapy must be coordinated with a specialist of infectious diseases [8].

PRIMARY CHRONIC OSTEOMYELITIS

According to **Bevin *et al.* in 2008**, Primary Chronic Osteomyelitis is that a straightforward disease to be managed easily. The varied treatments for Primary Chronic Osteomyelitis as dictated by **Vargas *et al.* in 1982** reflect the lack of understanding of the etiology of this disease. It is a chronic disease and despite aggressive surgical treatment, it shows recurrent behaviour [68].

According to **Paula *et al.* in 2009**, etiology of Primary Chronic Osteomyelitis is poorly understood [69]. The main goal of treatment in patients with primary chronic osteomyelitis must be to eliminate or at least ameliorate clinical symptoms since a cure cannot be guaranteed. Even though the disease may not yet be curable, change of course and severity should be considered [8].

According to Bevin *et al.* in 2008, the list of available treatment modalities in Primary Chronic Osteomyelitis is as follows [68]:

1. **Nonsurgical**: Antibiotics [108], Non Steroidal Anti-Inflammatory Drugs [108], Hyperbaric oxygen therapy [109], Bisphosphonate treatment [108 - 110] and Muscle relaxants [111].
2. **Surgical**: Decortications alone [109], Decortication with bone grafting [112], Partial (marginal) resection [113], and Segmental resection [108, 113].

Recently the nomenclature for this disease was discussed by **Eyrich *et al.* in 2003**. Using this nomenclature, primary chronic osteomyelitis is defined as chronic nonsuppurative osteomyelitis [68].

According to **Paula *et al.* in 2009**, as described previously, the course of early onset of primary chronic osteomyelitis known as Garre's osteomyelitis (juvenile chronic osteomyelitis) may differ from the adult type [69]. In addition, the stage of disease may be different in an earlier period as compared with a later stage.

According to **Bevin *et al.* in 2008**, in the decision-making process, the frequency of onset with pain, swelling, and limitation of mouth opening should be taken into account [68].

Therefore, according to **Baltensperger** *et al.* **in 2004**, the extent and aggressiveness of treatment may also differ. The large volume and extent of affected bone in most cases suggest complete surgical removal of the affected region as the best treatment option.

Jacobson *et al.* **in 1982** suggested an infectious etiology for primary chronic osteomyelitis.

Later **Marx in 1994** also confirmed the above findings.

But recently, in contrast to the above findings, according to **Paula** *et al.* **in 2009,** there is often a negative response to antibiotic treatment [69].

According to **Eyrich** *et al.* **in 1999** and **in 2003**, in the early stage of disease, operative procedures such as localized removal of all necrotic tissue and decortication are usually successful [21].

According to **Bevin** *et al.* **in 2008,** in an early stage of the disease with a large volume of altered bone with a high frequency of active periods, decortication corrects bone deformity, removes necrotic tissue, improves bony blood perfusion, and in most cases leads to a decrease in frequency of onset [68].

Bevin *et al.* **in 2008** further stated that decortication improves the blood supply owing to the fact that "the cortex" which acts as a barrier between rich blood supply of periosteum & surrounding soft tissue and the deeper marrow spaces [68].

According to **Eyrich** *et al.* **in 1999,** due to frequent involvement of reconstructed bone in PCO, resection and second-stage reconstruction should be considered carefully in later stages of the disease.

Further, according to **Eyrich** *et al.* **2003,** due to uncertain prognosis, excessive surgery should be avoided, especially in young patient population [21].

According to **Baltensperger in 2004**, conservative therapy plays an important role in patients with multiple unsuccessful interventions and elderly medically compromised patients. Conservative therapy involves hyperbaric oxygen therapy, non steroidal anti-inflammatory drugs, antibiotics, steroids, as well as bisphosphonates and other drugs [21].

According to **Baltensperger and Eyrich in 2000**, the overall role of hyperbaric oxygen therapy remains unclear in primary chronic osteomyelitis [8]. They further suggested that hyperbaric oxygen therapy is planned at twice daily sessions at 1.4 atmospheres for 45 minute cycles. It is carried out for a period of a minimum of 20 or more sessions. Further it is recommended that the antibiotics should be administered along with the hyperbaric oxygen therapy treatment [8].

According to **Bevin** *et al.* **in 2008**, patients of primary chronic osteomyelitis respond to administration of non-steroidal anti-inflammatory drugs with clearly reduced symptoms [68].

However, according to **Baltensperger and Eyrich in 2000,** during the course of disease, these non-steroidal anti-inflammatory drugs may become less effective [8].

Further, **Eyrich** *et al.* **in 1999** commented that in a long-standing therapy with non-steroidal anti-inflammatory drugs, side effects, such as gastro-intestinal and kidney problems must also be taken in to account.

According to **Eyrich** *et al.* **in 1999,** the steroids and the non-steroidal anti-inflammatory drugs block the inflammatory cascade on different mediatory levels. In long-standing refractory cases of diffuse osteomyelitis steroids may be considered, especially if the non-steroidal anti-inflammatory drugs are ineffective [8].

According to **Baltensperger in 2004,** a single dosage of 50 mg prednisone within 12 hours leads to immediate and complete relief of pain and swelling.

According to **Baltensperger and Eyrich in 2000**, patients treated with long-term antibiotic medication showed no, or at least a decreased frequency of mild symptoms while on medication. They further claimed that symptoms usually reoccur within 2 weeks after the last dosage of antibiotics is given [8]. The spectra of effective antibiotics are predominantly those targeting anaerobes, including clindamycine, amoxycillin, metranidazole, and tertracyclines.

Recently, several case reports by **Soubrier M** *et al.* **in 2001** and **Sugata** *et al.* **in 2003** reported favourable responses to pamidronate [108].

Lacassagne C *et al.* **in 2007** advocated the role of pamidronate along with other bisphosphonates.

According to **Yamazaki** *et al.* **in 2007,** both bone-specific alkaline phosphatase (bone formation marker) and pyridinoline cross-linked carboxyterminal telopeptide of type-I collagen (bone resorption marker) showed a marked decrease with pamidronate. It may therefore be useful in the treatment of primary chronic osteomyelitis due to its inhibitory effect on bone turnover.

According to **Baltensperger and Eyrich in 2000**, Pamidronate drug should be reserved to the patients who do not respond to the steroids or non-steroidal anti-inflammatory drugs.

According to **Lacassagne C *et al.* in 2007,** Pamidronate administration in patients with primary chronic osteomyelitis is only recommended in association with periods of onset for a short period. However, a mild reaction, such as low-grade fever and lassitude is well known. Hence, bisphosphonate-induced osteochemonecrosis of the jaws (Fig. **8.1**), as seen under long-term therapy, do not usually appear. Further, the therapy in young patients should be carefully considered because of its unknown teratogenic potential.

Overall, according to **Lacassagne C *et al.* in 2007,** Pamidronate seems to be an effective second-line therapy.

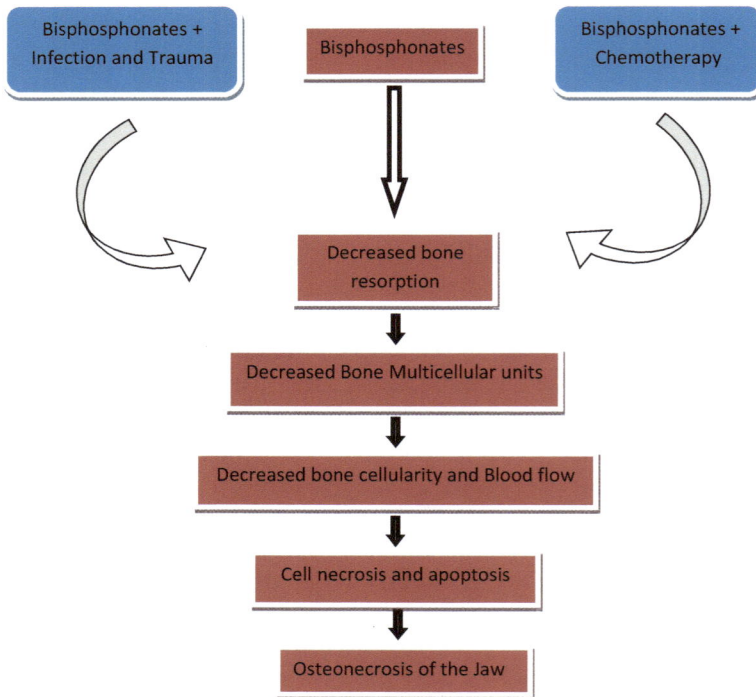

Fig. (8.1). Pathologic model for the development of osteonecrosis of the jaw due to Bisphosphonates according to **Migliorati *et al.* in 2005 [114]**.

According to **Eyrich in 1999,** in cases of syndrome-associated primary chronic osteomyelitis, treatment includes non-steroidal anti-inflammatory drugs while in refractory cases, administration of sufusalazine. Few persistent cases may require administration of methotrexate [8].

Diffuse Sclerosing Osteomyelitis

Successful treatment is generally dependent on correct diagnosis and should be based on available pathophysiological knowledge.

According to **Ogawa** *et al.* **in 2001**, diffuse sclerosing osteomyelitis causes diagnostic as well as therapeutic difficulties [112].

Unfortunately according to **Jacobsson in 1984**, the true nature of diffuse sclerosing osteomyelitis is obscure, so the treatment must be based on empirical findings [115].

According to **Jacobsson in 1984,** the most reasonable approach to this disease is a conservative one. The acute episodes can be treated by antibiotic administration, without any other intervention. Although the lesion may be slowly progressive, it is not particularly dangerous since it is not destructive and seldom produces complications [115].

According to **Kahn** *et al.* **in 1994**, the treatment of chronic diffuse sclerosing Osteomyelitis is a difficult problem [70]. Resolution of the adjacent foci of chronic infection often leads to improvement of the lesion [112].

But in contrast, according to **Ogawa** *et al.* **in 2001**, numerous treatments have been tried for chronic diffuse sclerosing Osteomyelitis including long term antibiotics as well as hyperbaric oxygen therapy. Unfortunately, the treatment for suspected infection often fails, even when combined treatment methods are used [112].

According to **Jacobsson in 1984,** if a tooth is present in the sclerotic areas and is required to be extracted, the probability of infection and protracted healing must be recognized. Sclerotic bone is hypovascular and responds poorly to any bacterial infection [115].

Bell has recommended tooth extraction as a last resort. It can be performed utilizing a surgical approach with removal of liberal amounts of bone to facilitate extraction and increased bleeding. Sclerosed bone may remain as such in some patients even after the resolution of the lesion and may be remodeled in others [50].

Various authors like **Jacobsson in 1984** and **Kahn** *et al.* **in 1994** advocated for antibiotic therapy for diffuse sclerosing osteomyelitis [70, 76] since a bacterial infection has been suspected. **Ogawa** *et al.* **in 2001** also supported this fact [112].

According to **Suei** *et al.* **in 1995**, decortication has been recommended [76] in order to improve the circulation by establishing contact between the periosteal vessels and the subcortical tissues, so that the body's natural defense mechanisms and antibiotics can better combat the infection. According to **Jacobsson in 1984**, hyperbaric oxygen therapy has been tried, since lowered oxygen tension and anaerobic infection are presumed [115].

According to **Jacobsson in 1984** and **Suei** *et al.* **in 1995**, Cortisone therapy was advocated [76, 155] because of the histological signs of vasculitis and the absence of common pathogenic organisms [76].

Garre's Osteomyelitis

According to **Felsberg in 1990**, it is defined as an intense proliferation of periosteum with reactive peripheral bone formation caused by a slight irritation or infection without necrosis or purulent exudates. Since **1893**, when **Carl Garré** described the features of the sclerosing osteomyelitis, few reports have been published [116].

According to **Martin-Granizo** *et al.* **in 1999**, this is a rather rare disease. It is also named periostitis ossificans, nonsuppurative chronic osteomyelitis, and chronic osteomyelitis with proliferative periostitis [116].

According to **Bell in 2006**, most cases of proliferative periostitis of the jaws are associated with periapical inflammatory lesions, and the treatment is extraction of the offending tooth or appropriate endodontic therapy directed toward eliminating the source of the infection [50, 117]. After the focus of infection has been eliminated and inflammation has resolved, the layers of the bone will consolidate in 6- 12 months as the overlying muscle action helps to remodel the bone in its original state.

According to **Martin-Granizo** *et al.* **in 1999,** if a unifocal periosteal reaction similar to proliferative periostitis appears in the absence of an obvious source of inflammation, biopsy is recommended [116]. This is so because according to **Felsberg** *et al.* **in 1990**, several neoplastic conditions like fibrous dysplasia, infantile cortical hyperostosis (Caffey's disease), Ewing's sarcoma, osteosarcoma, syphilitic osteomyelitis, hypertrophic osteoarthropathy, and even a healing fracture callus can result in a similar pattern [116].

According to **Malik in 2002**, the treatment modalities of Garre's osteomyelitis are directed towards removal of source of inflammation [16]. These are as follows:

S.No	Treatment
1	Removal of infected tooth and curettage of the extraction socket
2	Surgical recontouring to recontour the cortical expansion of the jaw
3	Endodontic therapy
4	Antibiotics if signs of infection are present
5	Follow up

Synovitis, Acne, Pustulosis, Hyperostosis, Osteitis (SAPHO) Syndrome

According to **Suei *et al*. in 2005**, most treatment directed towards elimination of infection in SAPHO syndrome has been proven ineffective [22].

According to **Kahn in 1994 and Suei *et al*. in 2005**, long-term antibiotic therapy has produced no noticeable results. Surgical decortication has decreased the intensity and frequency of symptoms but has failed to resolve the process totally [22, 70].

According to **Suei *et al*. in 1996,** steroidal and non-steroidal anti-inflammatory medications are reported to be the most effective agents to relieve symptoms, but they are usually associated with incomplete resolution [22, 24].

Suei *et al*. in 2005 further confirmed the above findings.

According to **Yoshii *et al*. in 2001**, long-term administration of macrolides is effective.

According to **van Merkesteyn in 1988**, muscle relaxation treatment methods have been reported to be effective.

According to **Suei *et al*. in 2005**, conservative treatment and long-term treatment with analgesics and antiinflammatory drugs have been recommended [22]. Recently, reports of treatment with pamidronate have given positive results. Even with significant surgical and medical interventions, the course is characterized by flares separated by partial remissions.

Chronic Recurrent Multifocal Osteomyelitis

According to **Suei *et al*. in 1994 and 1995**, the use of antimicrobial therapy with Chronic Recurrent Multifocal Osteomyelitis does not alter the course of the disease [75, 76].

According to **Suei *et al*. in 1995**, Nonsteroidal anti-inflammatory drugs such as naproxen, indomethacin or aspirin constitute initial treatment and a rapid course of corticosteroids is recommended in refractory cases. Nonsteroidal anti-inflammatory drugs which inhibit the cyclo-oxygenase 2, such as meloxicam, have been used in Chronic Recurrent Multifocal Osteomyelitis cases which do not respond to naproxen.

Other treatments such as sulfasalazine, methotrexate and a hyperbaric chamber, are indicated in painful and refractory cases.

According to **Stanton in 1993** and **Suei *et al.* in 1995** prognosis is doubtful with Chronic Recurrent Multifocal Osteomyelitis, which can present a prolonged and painful clinical course with intervals of inflammatory process activity and remission [76].

According to **Suei *et al.* in 1995,** goal of the treatment in Chronic Recurrent Multifocal Osteomyelitis should be alleviation of the symptoms while awaiting the resolution of the disease process [76].

According to **Otsuka K and Kayahara H in 1999**, it is important that pediatricians should recognize Chronic Recurrent Multifocal Osteomyelitis, and differentiate it from acute osteomyelitis avoiding prolonged and unnecessary antibiotic therapy [73].

According to **Otsuka K and Kayahara H in 1999,** Scintigraphy, tomography or magnetic resonance are useful to identify osteolytic lesions [73]. Biopsy is necessary in order to rule out bone tumors and infectious osteomyelitis. Initial treatment includes non-steroidal anti-inflammatory drugs and/or corticosteroids. A hyperbaric oxygen therapy or methotrexate can be used in refractory cases with significant or prolonged pain [73].

Management-Antibiotics

According to **Walker *et al.* in 1947**, early and adequate antibiotic therapy may lead to spontaneous resolution of the disease [9].

According to **Koorbusch *et al.* in 1992**, majority of the patients of osteomyelitis can be empirically treated with systemic antibiotics on an outpatient basis. He concluded that microbiologic cultures are not routinely required to direct antibiotic therapy [7].

Lew and Waldvogel in 1997 and 2004 advocated that the main treatment goal in osteomyelitis case is to support healing by completely eradicating microorganisms.

According to **Baltenspenger and Eyrich in 2000**, this goal is difficult to achieve in maxillofacial osteomyelitis. This was attributed to the presence of dentition as well as persistent exposure of bone to oral microorganisms. Henceforth pertinent and correct administration of microorganism directed antibiotics remains the mainstay of the osteomyelitis therapy [8].

Lazzarini *et al.* **in 2005** highlighted that there was optimism amongst the clinicians during the first decade of antibiotic era. This was attributed to marked clinical success in treatment of infectious diseases with the usage of antibiotics [96]. On the basis of this, few researchers like **Florey and Florey in 1943** made an opinion that surgery may not be required in osteomyelitis cases if antibiotics are administered at an early stage [96]. However this opinion was not successful due to huge record of clinical failure in few years in cases treated only with antibiotics.

By 1968, **Bick's book** highlighted review of 25 years of antibiotic treatment in osteomyelitic cases. This led the author to conclude that it is not valuable to treat osteomyelitis related septicemia and abscess with antibiotics alone. On the contrary surgical treatment of chronic bone infection is required to control the disease [8, 96].

Lazzarini *et al.* **in 2005** commented that there is sparse data regarding the effectiveness of antimicrobial agents used in osteomyelitis cases. There is still confusion regarding most effective antimicrobial agent, the duration as well as their route of administration in different types of osteomyelitis for best possible results [96]. Thus, the treatment of osteomyelitis is still mostly based on expert opinions and no consensus guidelines are currently available [96].

As already discussed above, duration of antibiotic therapy is crucial for the pertinent management of osteomyelitis. According to the papers reviewed regarding osteomyelitis from 1968 to 2001, majority of clinicians subjected the patients for six week of antibiotic therapy while a few followed six months regime too [96].

This is also in accordance with the treatment guidelines for acute and chronic osteomyelitis in adults recommended by **Johnston and Conly in 2007** which involved prolonged courses of antimicrobials, usually given intravenously [94].

According to **Lazzarini** *et al.* **in 2005**, 4-6 weeks of antibiotic therapy is recommended by all the clinicians for acute osteomyelitis cases [96]. On the contrary, according to **Johnston and Conly in 2007**, greater variability exists in the recommendation of the treatment of chronic osteomyelitis in terms of duration, route of administration, stage of infection and type of pathogen [94].

Data from animal models as shown by **Norden in 1988** reveal that bacteria can be cultured from infected bone even after two weeks of appropriate antibiotic therapy [118].

Waldvogel in 1988 advised that the usual antibiotic treatment for osteomyelitis must be four to six weeks [119].

Different types of osteomyelitis require different management strategies. According to **Lew and Waldvogel in 1997** and **2004**, antibiotics are a crucial pillar for the treatment of hematogenous osteomyelitis while surgery is usually not required or is limited to removal of foci of infection or debridement. This fact was in contrast to the findings of **Trampuz and Zimmerli in 2006** who reported that in cases of SCO, proper debridement or sequestrectomy is required for proper healing along with removal of necrotic bone. Furthermore, elimination of infective foci and dead-space management is also required on the basis of the location of the infection.

Nakajima *et al.* in 1977 described local implantation of antibiotic saturated beads in the treatment of osteomyelitis of the jaws.

Hudson in 1993 in his 50 year old prospective on osteomyelitis of jaws, described various methods to augment systemic host immune response to reach the site of infection. It includes:

i. Intra-arterial antibiotic therapy.
ii. Local implantation of antibiotic saturated beads.
iii. Hyperbaric Oxygen therapy.

Recommended Antibiotic Regimens for Osteomyelitis of Jaws [16]

1. **1ˢᵗ Choice**
    1. **Regimen I:** As empirical therapy, Penicillin V is given
        a. **Aqueous penicillin-** 2 million units IV every 4 hourly
        b. **Oxacillin-** 1 gm IV every 4 hourly
        When the patient has been asymptomatic for 48 to 72 hours, then switch to: Penicillin V orally 500 mg every 4 hourly with Cloxacillin 250 mg orally every 4 hourly for 2-4 weeks.
    2. **Regimen II:** It is based on culture and sensitivity results. Penicillinase-resistant penicillins, such as oxacillin, dicloxacillin, or flucloxacillin may be given.
        In case of allergy to penicillin, the following antibiotics are prescribed in order of preference
        i. Clindamycin 300-600 mg orally 6 hourly

    ii. Cephalosporin:
        a. Cefazolin 500 mg 8 hourly, or
        b. Cephalexin 500 mg 6 hourly
    iii. Erythromycin 2 mg every 6 hourly IV then 500 mg every 6 hourly orally.
2. **2nd Choice**
   Clindamycin: It is effective against penicillinase producing staphylococci, streptococci, and anaerobic bacteria including Bacteroids. It is used because of its ability to diffuse widely in bone. It is not recommended as a first choice as it is bacteriostatic and causes diarrhoea due to pseudomembranous colitis.
3. **3rd Choice**
   Cefazolin or Cephalexin: It is effective against most cocci including penicillinase producing staphylococci, Gram negative aerobic bacilli like *Klebsiella*, *E. Coli* and *Proteus*.
   Cephalosporins are not recommended as first choice because:
   i. These are moderately effective against anaerobes.
   ii. Because of broad spectrum coverage which increases antibiotic complications like bacterial resistance and superinfection.
4. **4th Choice**
   Erythromycin: These drugs cannot be used as first choice as these are bacteriostatic and rapidly develop resistant strains.
   The dose and duration of antimicrobial therapy is dependent upon severity of infection and its response to treatment.

Johnston and **Conly** reviewed several authoritative reviews on osteomyelitis which were published in **The New England Journal of Medicine in 2007** [94]. Some of those clinicians considered the selection of antibiotic on the basis of its reported penetration in the bone. This data of bony penetration of the antibiotics was derived from animal studies (rats or rabbits) in which the bone and serum concentration of antibiotics was experimentally assessed and measured.

The studies done by **Norden in 1989** and **Dworkin** *et al.* **in 1990** generally demonstrated excellent bone penetration by rifampicin while there was good penetration by fluoroquinolones also [120, 121]. **Mader** *et al.* **in 1989** highlighted that Clindamycin too demonstrated excellent bone penetration while Cefazolin demonstrated low bone concentration [122]. However multidrug resistant viridians group of streptococci (MDRVS) have emerged as important pathogens [122].

According to **Jocelyn in 2008,** Moxifloxacin appears to be an effective and attractive option for the treatment of MDRVS infections, including osteomyelitis [123].

Further, according to **Jocelyn in 2008,** Moxicillin is a fourth generation fluoroquinolone approved for the treatment of a variety of infections in adult patients [123]. In addition to its broad antibacterial activity against a variety of Gram-positive and Gram-negative bacteria, it has also been shown to have good activity against periodontal pathogens, including anaerobes and multidrug-resistant streptococci [123].

According to **Fritz *et al*. in 2009**, in some situations it may not be feasible to safely remove sequestrum or infected prosthetic material. In such cases, it may be necessary to prescribe oral antibiotics for long term suppression of infection [42].This therapy should be based on culture and susceptibility data.

Fritz *et al*. in 2009 further suggested that it is preferable to use agents that have good bioavailability in the maxillofacial region and can penetrate soft tissues as well [42].

Hence according to **Calhoun *et al*. in 2005** and **Fritz *et al*. in 2009,** quinolones, clindamycin and rifampicin are the attractive choices [42]. He further stated that because of cumulative risks of side effects, cumulative costs, and antibiotic resistance problems, suppressive antimicrobials should be avoided unless absolutely necessary [42].

Local Antibiotic Therapy: (According to Topazian in 2002) [1]

Closed Wound Irrigation-suction [1]

Tubes are placed against the bone to allow for drainage of pus and serum and to provide a route for irrigation in order to reduce the number of remaining microorganisms [1].

This type of therapy is especially helpful when determination of the extent of chronic infection of residual bone cannot be determined [1].

Irrigation without prior debridement is unlikely to be effective and it might actually prolong the process of infection.

Technique: According to **Topazian in 2002**, after debridement, saucerization or decortication, small pediatric nasogastric feeding tubes, French catheters or polyethylene irrigation tubes of 3-4mm in diameter and 6-10 inches in length are perforated along a distance 3-4 cm from the tip. The tubes are placed into the bone bed through separate skin incisions along the lateral bony surface and are affixed to the bone with sutures through holes drilled into the bone [1].

Two drains are usually placed, one serving for antibiotic irrigation while the second one for suction. The skin is closed watertight over the tubes [1].

Multiple ways of irrigation-suction system exist. Either 2 litres of antibiotic solution can be instilled and then suctioned every 24 hours or the solution can be instilled on a 12 hour cycle and left in place for 3 hours. It is then suctioned for 9 hours *via* a low intermittent suction.

Important points: The wound should not be overfilled and the volume of the irrigation antibiotic solution should be gradually decreased to allow for closure of the wound and healing [1].

Systemic antibiotics should be used throughout the irrigation period and at least for 2 months after the cessation of clinical evidence of disease [1].

Antibiotic – Impregnated Beads [1]

According to **Topazian in 2002**, the beads are used to deliver high concentrations of antibiotics into the wound bed and in immediate proximity to the infected bone. The beads release high local concentrations, but low systemic concentrations thus reducing the risk of toxicity.

According to **Topazian in 2002 and Coviello & Stevens in 2007**, Tobramycin, Gentamicin or Clindamycin is contained in acrylic resin (polymethylmeth acrylate) cement beads. Usually a chain of beads is applied against bleeding bone after decortication and a drain is inserted and the wound is closed. The system is left in place for 10-14 days [1, 30].

According to **Coviello & Stevens in 2007**, these local antibiotic delivery systems are of two types. They may be nonresorbable or resorbable [30].

According to Coviello & Stevens in 2007, advantages of resorbable local antibiotic delivery systems over the nonresorbable delivery systems are as follows:

  i. They do not require second surgery for removal.
 ii. Low-grade foreign body reactions are uncommon in contrast to nonresorbable antibiotic delivery system.
iii. They have a predictable local release of antibiotics.

Hence, according to **Nelson *et al.* in 2002**, Biodegradable antibiotic delivery materials are therefore an attractive concept in the development of local antibiotic delivery systems [124].

According to **Topazian in 2002**, systemic antibiotics should be administered simultaneously [1].

Management-Surgical Treatment

The surgical procedures used to treat osteomyelitis have been adequately described in the literature by **Khosla in 1970, Glahn in 1974** and **Sanders in 1978 [7]**. Surgical treatment was later described by **Koorbusch *et al.* in 1992, Momenten in 1993, Flygare *et al.* in 1997** and **Ogawa *et al.* in 2001.**

It was further explored in detail by **Yeoh in 2005, Bevin *et al.* in 2008** and **Ducic in 2008**.

According to **Topazian RG in 2002**, surgical intervention is usually an adjunct to medical management [1].

According to **Johnston and Conly in 2007,** it is the mainstay of treatment in chronic osteomyelitis [94]. In the acute stage it should be limited to removal of severely loose teeth and bone fragments and incision and drainage of fluctuant areas. This may proceed to sequestrectomy with or without saucerization, decortication, resection and then reconstruction [1].

Most of the authors like **Topazian RG in 2002**, support surgical intervention under antibiotic coverage at least 1-2 days prior to the procedure [1].

In contrast some authors like **Lazzaraini *et al.* in 2002 & 2004** and **Baltensperger & Eyrich in 2000** prefer antibiotic sensitivity testing to be performed [8, 96].

Surgical Procedures Involved Include the Following:

Incision and Drainage

According to **Adekeye *et al.* in 1985,** establishment of suppuration essentiates the need for surgical drainage [9].

According to **Malik in 2002**, incision and drainage should be done as soon as possible. It relieves the pressure and pain caused by the accumulation of pus [16].

Further, according to **Malik in 2008**, evacuation of pus by drainage lessens the absorption of toxic products and prevents further spread of infection in the bone, thus helping in its localization [16].

According to **Topazian in 2002**, unless the abscess is extensive or pus is located deeply, the initial drainage and debridement may be accomplished with the patient under local anaesthesia and sedation. Deeply located or extensive abscesses may require treatment with the patient under general anaesthesia. Heat should be avoided in such cases because it may encourage extension of infection through bone [1].

According to Malik NA in 2008, methods employed for drainage includes [16]:

a. Opening up of the pulp chamber.
b. Making fenestration through the cortical plate over the apical area with a drill.
c. In an edentulous area, especially posterior maxilla or tuberosity region, pus is removed by making an incision over the alveolar crest and by making a window.
d. At the angle of the mandible or ascending ramus, drainage can be achieved by a small incision made over a point of greatest tenderness or just below the mandible.

The consistency, colour and odour of the pus may provide important clues to the diagnosis and initial treatment.

Extraction of Loose or Offending Tooth

According to **Topazian in 2002**, extraction of the carious teeth with periapical infection in the concerned area with periapical infection should be done [1]. Sometimes the drainage can be done by mere extraction of the offending tooth only.

Mowlem in 1945 considered paradoxical tooth extraction implicated in the treatment of osteomyelitis [9].

However, **Archer in 1975** stressed the importance of extracting those teeth which have lost their bony support [9].

Debridement

According to **Baltensperger and Eyrich in 2000**, thorough debridement of the affected area should be carried out after incision and drainage [8, 16].

According to **Malik in 2002**, after thorough debridement, the area may be irrigated with hydrogen peroxide and saline. Any foreign body or necrotic tissue should be removed [16].

But according to **Fritz in 2009,** one stage approach with debridement alone is less likely to achieve cure [42].

Sequestrectomy

According to **Topazian in 2002**, sequestra can be cortical, cancellous or cortico-cancelous and are usually seen after 2 weeks from the onset of the infection [1].

According to **Adekeye** *et al.* **in 1985**, sequestrectomy is mandatory if sequestra are formed (Figs. **8.2-8.6**) [9]. Once they get fully formed, they can persist for several months before they are resorbed, removed, or spontaneously expelled through the mucosa or the skin [16].

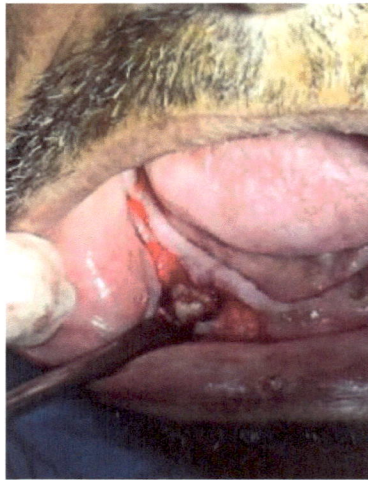

Fig. (8.2). Bony sequestra exposed in the mandibular alveolar ridge.

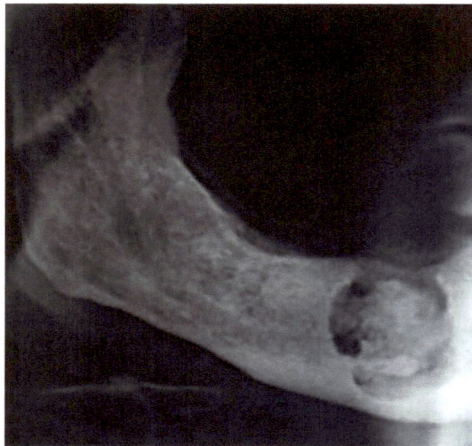

Fig. (8.3). Cropped OPG of the same patient revealing sequestra in the body of the mandible.

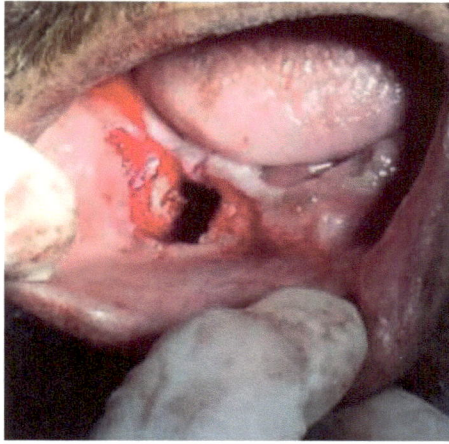

Fig. (8.4). Post surgery photograph after sequestractomy.

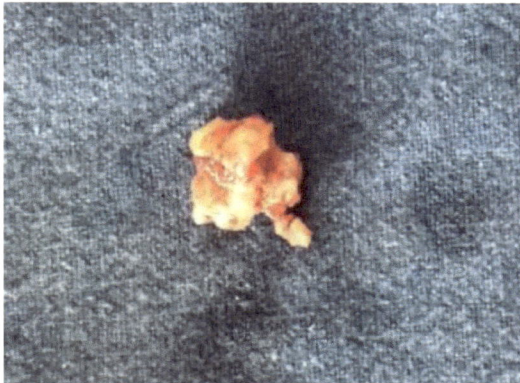

Fig. (8.5). Sequestrea removed from the patient's mandible.

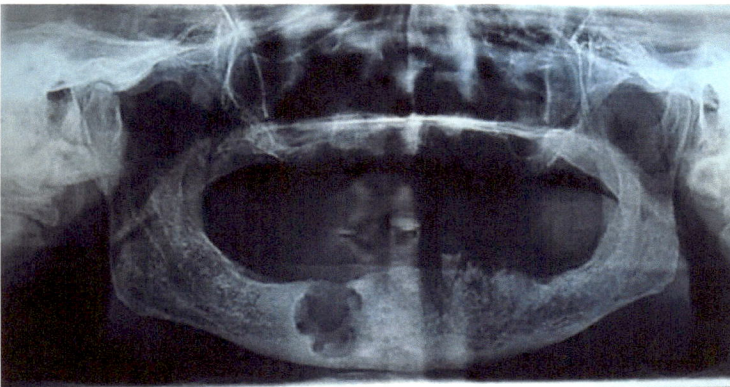

Fig. (8.6). Post operative OPG of the same patient.

According to **Malik in 2002**, the lytic activity of osteoclastic cells leads to the resorption of sequester. Later there is in growth of granulation tissue into the sequester promoting its degradation [16].

According to **Khosla in 1970**, being avascular, the sequestra are therefore poorly penetrated by antibiotics.

Adekeye *et al*. in 1985 also stressed upon the importance of timing of removal of the sequestra [9].They concluded that sequestra should be removed when fully formed.

Further, **Adekeye *et al*. in 1985** also supported the findings suggested by **Archer in 1975** according to which curettage to loosen a sequestrum should be avoided. This was attributed to the fact that there is destruction of delicate granulation tissue barrier between the normal bone and the sequestrum due to early intervention [9]. This leads to further extension of infection by shifting the balance between healing and breakdown [9]. Furthermore, the infection may even disseminate into blood stream resulting in septicemia too [9].

According to **Baltensperger and Eyrich in 2000**, the body tries to isolate the sequester in untreated or insufficiently treated cases of SCO. Periosteum produces a shell of bone known as involucrum. This involucrum serves as a barrier and is perforated by tracts known as cloacae. These cloacae let the pus drain to the epithelial surfaces. Larger sequestrum highlights instability of the jaw in terms of strength and may lead to pathological fractures.

Saucerization

This is considered as a further extensive surgical step followed during the surgical debridement of infected jawbone.

Baltensperger and Eyrich in 2000 mentioned this procedure as surgical "unroofing" of the jawbone. This will lead to exposure of the infected medullary cavity of the affected bone with osteomyelitis and will aid in subsequent thorough debridement [8].

Topazian in 2002 also supported the above mentioned fact [1].

According to Malik in 2002, saucerization allows direct access to already formed and forming sequestra, granulation tissue, and affected bone [16].

According to **Baltensperger and Eyrich in 2000**, the affected alveolar nerve may also be addressed in a limited fashion [16].

However, in cases of advanced acute and secondary chronic osteomyelitis with significant granulation tissue surrounding the inferior alveolar nerve, the created access by saucerization is insufficient [8]. According to **Topazian in 2002**, the saucerization procedure when performed by oral approach provides direct access to the jaw bone and hence there will be no extraoral scarring [1].

On the contrary, **Baltensperger and Eyrich in 2000** considered oral approach to be more challenging since it is difficult to collect non-contaminated specimen suitable for microbiological investigation [8].

Saucerization can be useful in early acute osteomyelitis cases and cases of limited extent. In early stages of the infection it leads to decompression of the medullary cavity. This decompression is advantageous as it allow extrusion of pus, debris, granulation tissue, and avascular fragments [8].

Saucerization of the Mandible (Modified After Topazian 2002)

a. A mucoperiosteal flap is raised by a gingival crest incision and access to bone is achieved.
b. There should be minimal reflection of the flap so as to preserve local blood supply.
c. Any mobile and affected teeth and other foci present in the affected area are removed.
d. Reduction of the lateral cortex of the mandible is achieved with the help of burs and rongeurs until bleeding bone is encountered at all the margins that too up to the level of the unattached mucosa. This will produce a saucer like defect.
e. Local debridement is performed. This includes removal of granulation tissue as well as loose bone fragments from the bone bed with the help of curettes.
f. Irrigation of the debrided area is thoroughly performed with the help of sterile saline solution with or without additional antibiotics such as Neomycin.
g. A medicated pack may be placed so as to provide local compression in case there is substantial local bleeding due to hyperaemia caused due to inflammatory process.
h. The trimmed buccal flap is then covered with medicated packs such as iodoform gauze with antibiotic and local steroid ointment for haemostasis and to maintain the flap in a retracted position. The pack is placed firmly without pressure. Retention of the flap is achieved by several nonresorbable sutures extending over the pack from the lingual to the buccal flap.
i. The pack is kept in place for several days and maximum up to 2-3 weeks. It may also be replaced several times until the surface of the bed of granulation tissue is epithelized and the margins have healed.

Decortication

Obwegeser in 1960 was the first person to carry out decortication procedure [68].

According to **Baltensperger and Eyrich in 2000**, decortication refers to the removal of chronically infected cortex of bone [8].

According to **Malik in 2002**, the lateral and inferior border cortex is removed 1 to 2 cm beyond the affected area thus providing access to the medullary cavity [8, 16].

Decortication was first advocated for jaw osteomyelitis by **Mowlem** in **1917.** He further advocated decortication in the treatment of osteomyelitis of the jaws in his studies. It has also been well described in the antibiotic era.

The application of this surgical procedure in conjunction with antibiotic therapy was later well described by **Obwegeser in 1960** and **Hjorting-Hansen in 1970**. The decortication procedure quickly became an established and widespread procedure for surgical osteomyelitis therapy [8].

According to **Obwegeser in 1960**, decortication procedure shortens the healing time. It was further supported by **Malik in 2002** and **Bevin in 2008** [16, 68].

According to **Topazian in 2002**, in advanced acute and secondary chronic osteomyelitis of the jaws, especially of the mandible, use of decortications promote resolution provided the affected cortical bone is avascular and harbours microorganisms [1]. Further the medullary cavity of the affected bone must show destruction with replacement by granulation tissue and pus.

Malik in 2002 highlighted that parenteral or orally administered antibiotics are not of much use as they cannot reach the affected region. Waiting for sequester formation and reducing surgery to sequestrectomy is not an option because of the advanced stage of the infection with risk for further spread, abscess formation, and cellulitis.

Furthermore, according to **Baltensperger and Eyrich in 2000**, the disadvantages associated with prolonged antibiotic therapy may become more prominent with time [8].

According to **Bevin *et al.* in 2008**, the major purpose of the decortication procedure is to remove the chronically infected cortex of the jawbone and gain access to affected medullary cavity to allow a sufficient decompression of intramedullary pressure and meticulous surgical debridement under direct visualization [68].

Bevin *et al.* in 2008 further stated that this procedure enhances the blood supply to the marrow as the cortex of the bone which acts as a barrier between rich blood supply of the periosteum and the deeper marrow spaces is removed [68].

Furthermore, according to **Bevin *et al.* in 2008**, this procedure allows bringing well-perfused tissue *e.g.,* masseter muscle in contact with bone thus, promoting further healing [68].

Montonen *et al.* in 1993 also evaluated decortication procedure and eventually performed 61 decortications [68].

The decortication procedure was originally described as a procedure with an extraoral approach. On the contrary **Bevin *et al.* in 2008** supported the intraoral approach to prevent facial scarring [68].

At the **Department of Cranio-Maxillofacial Surgery in Zurich**, which was founded by **Hugo Obwegeser**, the intraoral approach has been used whenever possible since the introduction of this procedure.

Baltensperger in 2003 also followed the philosophy of **Obwegeser** which is reflected by his reviewed data of 173 decortication procedures performed on osteomyelitis cases by an intraoral access from **1970 to 2000 [8]**. He also concluded that intraoral approach should be used whenever possible for decortication procedures.

Trephination or Fenestration

According to **Malik in 2002,** it is the creation of bony holes or windows in the overlying cortical bone adjacent to the infectious process for the tissue ammoniation and decompression of the medullary compartment [16].

According to **Baltensperger in 2003**, drilling of the holes into the cortex and reaching medulla provide multiple surgical transcortical ports that allow vascular communication between the periosteum and medullary cavity.

Resection

According to **Topazian in 2002** and **Malik in 2002,** when extensive portion of the bone is involved in the disease process, then resection of the jaw bone is advocated [16].

Baltensperger in 2003 and 2004 also supported the above mentioned fact.

According to **Topazian in 2002,** bone is debrided using an extraoral approach until bleeding surfaces are encountered distally and proximally [1]. This technique has been used successfully in cases of pathological fracture, persistent infection after decortications and marked disease of both cortical plates [1].

Immediate and/or Delayed Reconstruction

According to **Baltensperger & Eyrich in 2000 and Malik in 2002**, reconstruction is advocated following resection [16]. This is so as to

a. To maintain the continuity of the fragments.
b. To prevent pathological fracture
c. To prevent facial deformity
d. To provide attachment of the soft tissues.

Topazian in 2002 advocated that resection of the osteomyelitic area with immediate or delayed reconstruction may be necessary to resolve the low-grade and persistent chronic osteomyelitis [1].

According to **Topazian in 2002**, for immediate reconstruction, single or multiple blocks of autologous corticocancellous bone grafts are secured to a reconstruction plate. Particulate cancellous bone graft material is packed around the plate, split ribs forming a crib are packed with cancellous bone and wired into place [1].

According to **Malik in 2002**, the Illiac crest is a desirable graft. A block of corticocancellous iliac crest can be used or cancellous marrow can be used. Stabilization may be achieved with Vitallium or Titanium mesh that also serves as a tray to contain the graft. Immediate reconstruction offers the obvious advantage of shortening the period of illness and speeding recovery and rehabilitation. In cases where immediate bone grafting is contraindicated, a reconstruction plate can be used as a spacer [16].

CHAPTER 9

Critical Analysis and Discussion

Abstract: Besides discussing the osteomyelitis of the jaws, this particular chapter highlights the analysis of classification system as well as analysis of certain older terms regarding osteomyelitis which have been used in the literature. As it is well understood that Zurich system of classification has various advantages as compared to other different classification systems used in the literature, there still exist certain older terms for osteomyelitis which are actually misnomers. These include Condensing Osteitis and Focal sclerosing Osteomyelitis. Further, there are certain other rare types of osteomyelitis in which it is very difficult to trace the actual reason or causative agent. Those kinds of osteomyelitis may have a separate position in the classification system. One such example is tuberculous osteomyelitis in which sometimes it becomes difficult to trace the cause.

Keywords: Condensing Osteitis, Diffuse sclerosing osteomyelitis, Focal Sclerosing osteomyelitis, Mandible, Maxilla, Radiographic sclerosis, Trabeculae, Tuberculous Osteomyelitis, Zurich system of classification of Osteomyelitis of jaws.

CRITICAL ANALYSIS

Apart from the fact that there are several advantages of the Zurich system of classification of osteomyelitis of the jaws as has been described and followed in this book, there are certain old terminologies which still remain in the dark.

This includes **Condensing Osteitis** or **Focal Sclerosing Osteomyelitis**.

Holly D *et al.* in 2009 highlighted that condensing osteitis is a reaction of the bone to infection. This reaction leads to bone formation in contrast to bone destruction as seen in other periapical inflammatory diseases resulting in a radiopaque lesion. This is further attributed to low virulence of the offending microorganism coupled with good patient's resistance towards infection. Younger age group is frequently affected with this lesion with a predilection for periapical region of mandibular molars. It is seen to be associated with a carious tooth or a tooth with a large restoration. Some authors believed that the knowledge regarding the involvement of pulp as a causative factor in Condensing Osteitis is not complete as involvement of pulp is not necessary for condensing osteitis to happen. However current level of knowledge suggests that the involvement of pulp by carious lesion is mandatory for the disease to happen [125]. In contrast to pulpal degeneration, sometimes a pulpally sound tooth with periodontal problem is also believed to initiate condensing osteitis.

Etiology

Infection of periapical tissues by organisms of low virulence.

Clinical Features

As discussed above, condensing osteitis mostly occurs in younger individuals in mandibular molar tooth that too before 20 years of age.

Following are the presenting clinical features in condensing osteitis:

i. Clinically the teeth presents with big carious lesion involving pulp. In other words, the associated tooth is non-vital or with pulp undergoing the process of degeneration.
ii. Such teeth are usually asymptomatic. In some cases, the tooth may be tender on percussion or palpation.

Radiographic Appearance

It presents as a localized radiopaque lesion at the periapical region surrounding the affected tooth. The size, extent and margins of the lesion are variable. The margins vary from well defined to ill defined. There may be narrowing of inferior dental canal due to sclerosis. Hence it is obvious that a clinical diagnosis is very difficult in such cases. Radiographic sclerosis at the apex of the tooth root can be a clue to the diagnosis. Laboratory investigations can show an area of dense bone with trabeculae lined by osteoblasts. Chronic inflammatory cells, plasma cells and lymphocytes are also seen in scanty bone marrow.

Treatment

As per protocol, only those cases are treated which are symptomatic. The treatment includes endodontic therapy or extraction. Asymptomatic cases are kept on follow up. Those asymptomatic cases with no evidence of carious lesion in the associated tooth are examined and kept on follow up by periodic X ray examination.

Prognosis

The lesion of condensing osteitis remains in the jaws for indefinite time in case the offending tooth associated with it is extracted.

Differential Diagnosis

Hypercementosis, Osteosclerosis and cementoblastoma.

An abnormal result with electric pulp testing strongly suggests condensing osteitis and tends to rule out osteosclerosis and cementoblastoma.

Hence, according to this discussion, it is obvious that there is a source of infection involved in condensing osteitis and the occurrence of the disease is of long duration. So it must fall under **secondary chronic osteomyelitis**. But on the contrary, according to **Eyrich and Baltensperger in 2003**, in Zurich system, the term 'Secondary chronic osteomyelitis' is reserved for suppuratve osteomyelitis while **Primary chronic osteomyelitis** is defined as chronic nonsuppurative osteomyelitis. So as the condensing osteomyelitis is nonsuppurative, it also fulfils the criteria of Primary chronic osteomyelitis. However it should be noted that in chronic osteomyelitis, the etiology is ill defined.

So this can be regarded as a disadvantage of Zurich system of classification.

Furthermore there must be a separate provision for **Tuberculous osteomyelitis** in the **Zurich system of classification**. This disease is categorized under secondary chronic osteomyelitis in the **Zurich system of classification** but according to **Sheikh and Gupta *et al.* in 2012,** diagnosing tuberculous osteomyelitis is sometimes cumbersome. Because there is no clear etiological factor involved sometimes, it remains as a dilemma as all the clinical features as well as the laboratory tests required to confirm tuberculosis may prove to be negative. So the treatment is more of trial method [126].

Discussion

Historically osteomyelitis was a good topic of debate amongst various clinicians like **Caldwel and Goodwin in 1990's** because of its wide incidence, high percentage of mortality & morbidity and its economic importance to the society [43].

It is interesting to note that there is nothing in the ancient medical or dental literature regarding osteomyelitis until **J.L. Petit** described an acute infection of the bone in the **early part of eighteenth century** which corresponds to what is known as osteomyelitis now a days [42]. Although there is drastic reduction in the reported cases of osteomyelitis of the jaws due to the introduction of chemotherapeutic and antibiotic agents, this particular disease is still responsible for significant pain and suffering in the present [38]. To some extent, it is attributed to the fact that dental professionals are not able to recognise osteomyelitis of the jaws at an early stage of the disease.

As discussed earlier in this book, Osteomyelitis is an inflammatory condition of the bone. It begins as an infection of the medullary spaces and extends to involve the periosteum of the affected area.

As advocated by **Hoen** *et al.* **in 1988**, this infection later becomes established in the cortical portion of the bone. This further leads to local ischemia and eventual necrosis [38].

It is known to be a bacterial disease and mandible is by far most frequently affected site. Still some cases of osteomyelitis do not present with a clear etiology. Various classifications of osteomyelitis have been established based on clinical course, pathologic-anatomic or radiologic features, etiology, and pathogenesis. Unfortunately according to **Eyrich** *et al.* **in 2003**, a mixture of these classification systems has occurred throughout the literature. This has lead to confusion and has thereby hindered comparative studies in the field.

Further, there was a huge controversy in the literature regarding the time frame of conversion of acute osteomyelitis to chronic. **Marx in 1994** [71, 99] and **Mercuri in 1991** [52] clearly elaborated an arbitrary time of 1 month after the onset of initial symptoms for the conversion of acute osteomyelitis to chronic [21]. This chronic osteomyelitis may become suppurative with the formation of abscess or fistula. It may also present with sequestration at some stage of the disease [21]. At this stage, it is known as Secondary chronic osteomyelitis.

On the contrary, it may present as a nonsuppurative chronic inflammation with unknown etiology known as Primary chronic osteomyelitis [126 - 128].

The term *diffuse sclerosing osteomyelitis* (DSO) has been used as a broad nonspecific term and therefore may cause confusion. Different authors have used the term to describe different disease processes [21]. It merely describes a radiologic appearance that can be caused by several different entities such as Primary Chronic Osteomyelitis, Secondary Chronic Osteomyelitis, chronic tendoperiostitis, and ossifying periostitis (Garre's osteomyelitis).

According to the recent nomenclature given by **Eyrich** *et al.*, PCO when occurs in children and adolescents in known as Garre's osteomyelitis.

Osteoradionecrosis, which was once thought of as a radiation induced osteomyelitis (radio-osteomyelitis), has conclusively been identified as a radiation-induced avascular necrosis of bone [21, 71, 99] and therefore according to **Marx in 1983**, it should not be regarded as a form of osteomyelitis.

Imaging modalities are vital for the diagnosis and follow up in the case of osteomyelitis of the jaws [38]. As already discussed, there exists a wide variety of osteomyelitis which necessitates the application of different imaging techniques so as to achieve an accurate diagnosis [38, 128 - 131]. These imaging modalities are advised based on the clinical presentation of the disease and the experience of the dental professional. Most of the clinicians and researchers advocate Conventional radiography as the first imaging modality to start with [38] so as to have an overview of the normal anatomy and pathologic conditions of the bone and soft tissues of the region of interest. Ultrasonography is considered useful in the diagnosis of fluid collections, periosteal involvement, and surrounding soft tissue abnormalities. Many a time the clinicians advocate ultrasonography as it is helpful in providing guidance for diagnostic or therapeutic aspiration, drainage, or tissue biopsy [38]. Computed tomography scan can be advised to highlight osseous erosion at an early stage. It can also prove useful to document the presence of sequestrum, foreign body, or gas formation. However, it is found to be less sensitive to detect infection in the bone as compared to MRI. Magnetic resonance imaging is the most sensitive and most specific imaging modality for the detection of osteomyelitis and provides superb anatomic detail and more accurate information of the extent of the infectious process and soft tissues involved. Nuclear medicine imaging is particularly useful in identifying multifocal osseous involvement [38].

There are different varieties of osteomyelitis as highlighted in the section of classifications of the disease. Henceforth, there are different treatment protocols for different types. On the contrary, one common protocol for all the subtypes is to achieve a shift in the disturbed balance between the responsible pathogen(s) and host defences to normal [8]. This will allow the body to overcome the infection. Surgical removal of the infected bone and other associated necrotic tissue along with administration of antibiotics will lead to reduction in the number of pathogens. It is well known that Osteomyelitis leads to hindrance in vascularity and further the necrotic tissues do not let the antibiotics reach the target region. Henceforth a sufficient surgical debridement along with surgical decortication leads to improvement in local vascularization and promotes healing by bringing well-vascularized tissue in contact with the affected bone in cases of advanced acute and secondary chronic osteomyelitis of jaws [8]. It also facilitates the antibiotics to reach the target area in sufficient amount [8]. Therefore, surgery and antibiotics are to be considered the major columns in treating osteomyelitis of the jaws. The extent of surgical debridement depends upon the anatomical amount of bony involvement on the basis of imaging modality advocated.

After reviewing a lot of studies regarding treatment, it was concluded that the available literature on the treatment of osteomyelitis with antibiotics is inadequate to determine the best agents, route or duration of antibiotic therapy [21, 36]. This is also in accordance with the findings of **Stengel** *et al.* **in 2001, Lazzaraini** *et al.* **in 2005, Johnston and Conly in 2007 [36].**

Further, special emphasis should be paid on the systemic diseases leading to osteomyelitis. This includes Tuberculous osteomyelitis, Crohn's disease and deep fungal infections. After reviewing such a vast literature on osteomyelitis, it was observed that such reported cases are extremely rare in the dental and medical literature. However, the occurrence of such diseases is not that rare. This illustrates that these cases often go unnoticed by the dental as well as medical professionals. Obviously the sufferer will be the patient. Hence an expertise is required in diagnosing such cases. There was a similar case of tuberculous involvement of mandibular condyle in whom tuberculosis was suspected later. In this case the role of diagnostic techniques was emphasized as the osteomyelitis of condyle has the risk of being easily missed due to its atypical signs and symptoms and atypical radiographic appearance [126].

Tuberculous involvement of the mandibular condyle is very rare and only few such cases are reported so far [126], one in **Oral Surgery Oral Medicine Oral Pathology and Endodontology** in **1998,** one in **British Dental Journal** in **2003** and one in Dentomaxillofacial Radiology in 2012 in the literature [126]. Further the diagnosis of such a case is extremely difficult as there are no specific signs pathognomic of infections. The only manifestation may be a localized painful swelling of the jaw [126]. So, sometimes there are only trial based methods which have to be approached for the early treatment of such cases.

It is concluded that diagnosing osteomyelitis of the jaws and hence the treatment is a combination of art and science. It is rightly highlighted by **Johnston BL** and **Conly JM** in **2007** that the art of dentistry appears to play a role in continued fashion for the diagnosis and treatment, with science providing some foundation [36]. Since osteomyelitis of the jaws is a recognized heterogeneous infection; it is still difficult to believe non-availability of better human trials to guide investigation and treatment [36].

APPENDIX

Appendix: Radiographs and Imaging of Osteomyelitis of Jaws
By Dr. John KM Aps

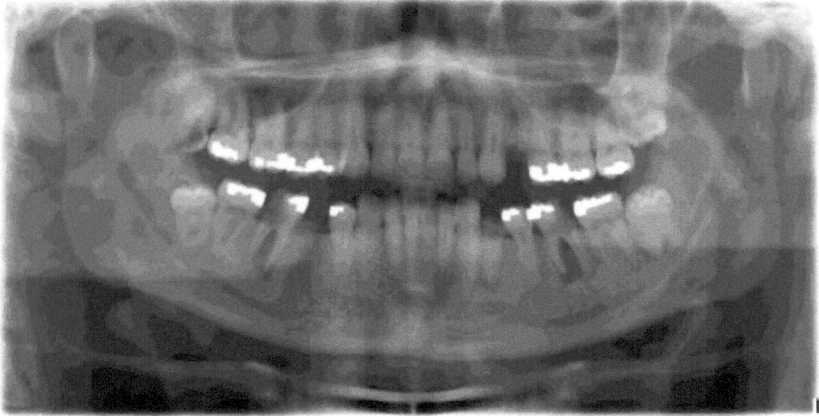

Fig. (A.1). Bilateral osteomyelitis with right ramus involvement.

DESCRIPTION

The increased density of the cancellous bone is obvious throughout the entire mandible and in the right mandibular ramus. The alveolar socket of the extracted mandibular premolar and the periapical infections at the right and left first molar and the left first premolar have ignited the bone to respond by diffuse sclerosis.

A.2 a

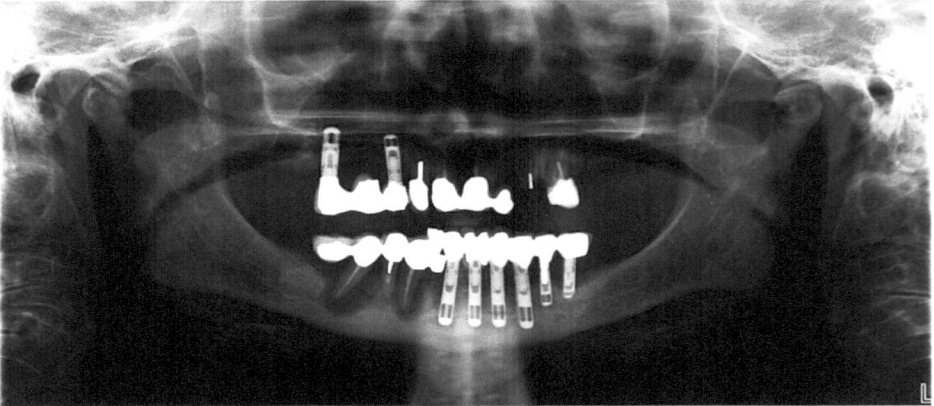

A.2 b

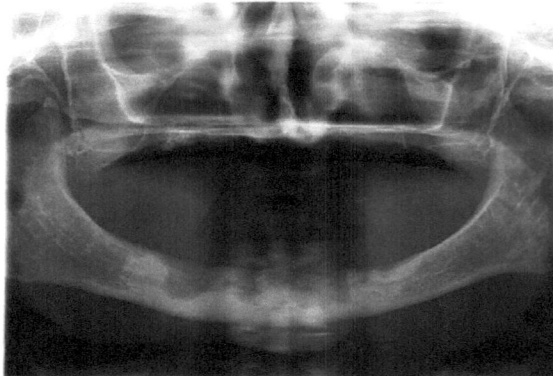

Fig. (A.2). Osteomyelitis anterior mandible after extractions.

DESCRIPTION

The image at the top shows the patient with several large infections on the right side of the mandible, at the apices of the canine and the premolars. It was considered best for the patient to have all remaining teeth extracted and to remove all of the implants. In the image at the bottom, one can see the ragged moth eaten radiolucent patches on the right side of the mandible with inferior denser sclerotic bone. The sclerotic bone formation is typical in chronic osteomyelitis.

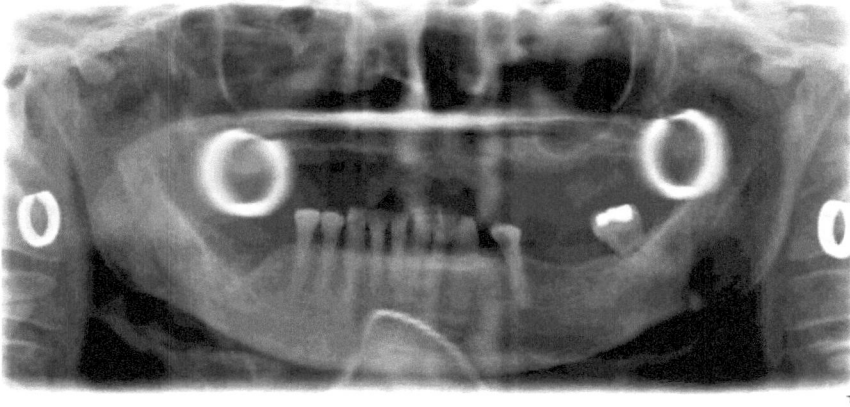

Fig. (A.3). Osteomyelitis DDX osteonecrosis bisphosphonate therapy and dental extraction.

DESCRIPTION

This patient had bisphosphonate intravenous therapy for breast cancer with bone metastases. Subsequent extraction of the second right mandibular molar caused a purulent wound in the mouth with bone sequesters being exposed recurrently. This panoramic radiograph was taken 6 months after the extraction. Osteomyelitis continued to bother the patient and bone sequesters kept appearing even after hyperbaric oxygen therapy, interventional surgery and numerous antibiotic treatments.

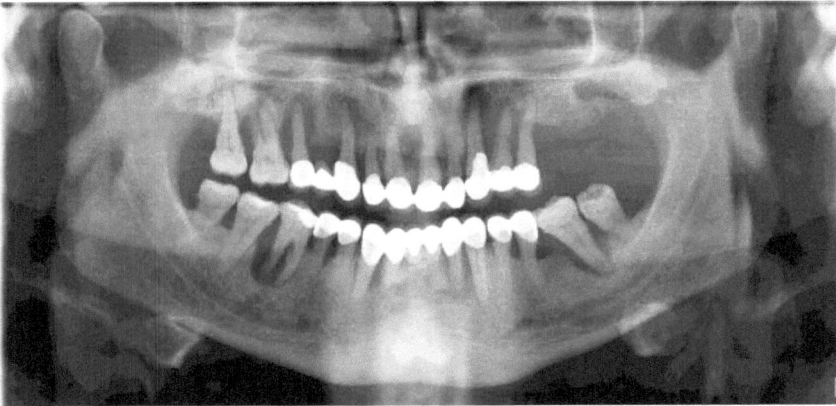

Fig. (A.4). Osteomyelitis in maxilla bilaterally.

DESCRIPTION

Surrounding the radiolucent periodontal lesions in the maxilla and the mandible, one can observe the diffuse osteosclerosis which is typical for chronic osteomyelitis.

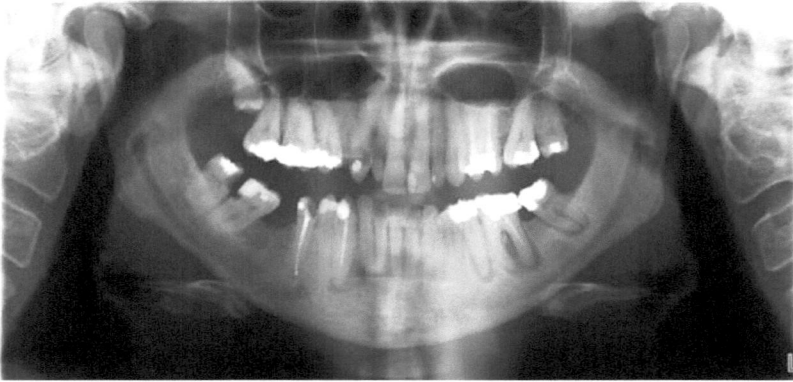

Fig. (A.5). Osteomyelitis left side of mandible into ramus.

DESCRIPTION

From the right second mandibular premolar into the left side of the body of the mandible one can appreciate the denser character of the trabecular pattern in the cancellous bone as a reaction to the three radiolucent lesions associated with the right canines, the left second premolar, the left first molar and the left third molar. The osteosclerosis appears to reach all the way up into the left ramus of the mandible.

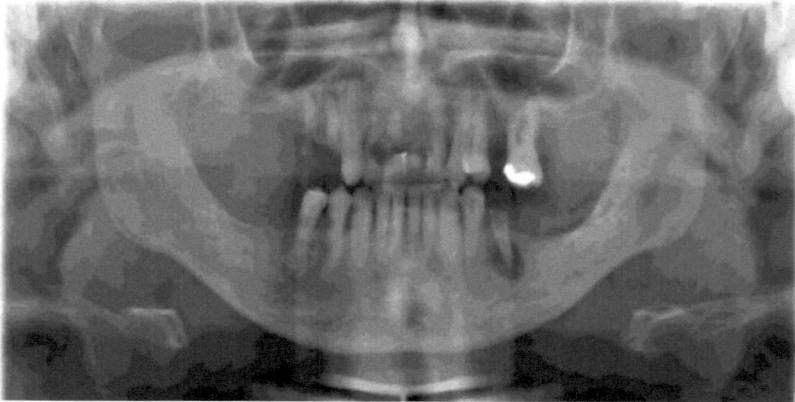

Fig. (A.6). Osteomyelitis left side of mandible.

DESCRIPTION

On the left side of the body of the mandible, one can appreciate a well defined, not corticated, uniform radiolucent, lesion which is surrounded by denser packed cancellous bone. This is typical osteosclerosis. Also notice that the left inferior alveolar canal is more apparent than the right canal, due to the increased density of the cancellous bone on the left side.

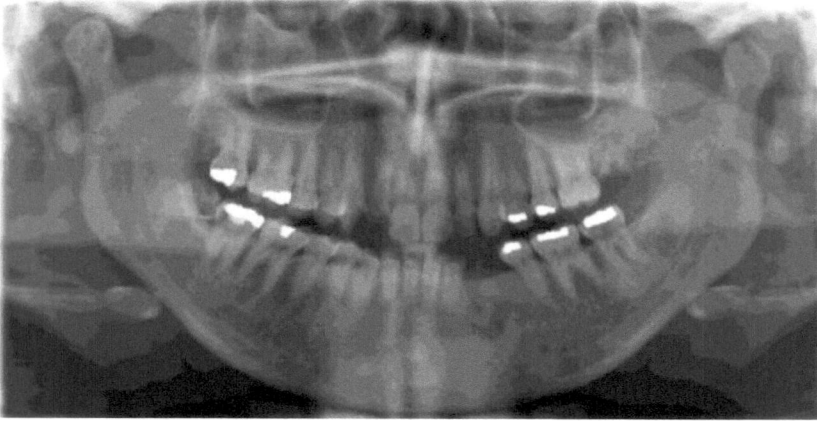

Fig. (A.7). Osteomyelitis left with sequester.

DESCRIPTION

The left side of the body of the mandible shows an extraction site of the canine, with a bony sequester in the radiolucent lesion where the apex of the canine used to be. Surrounding the radiolucent lesion is sclerosis of bone visible.

In the left side of the maxilla another osteomyelitis lesion is observed at the root fragments of the second molar. Notice how the floor of the maxillary sinus is affected and that the cortical border of the floor of the sinus has disappeared due to sclerosis of the bone.

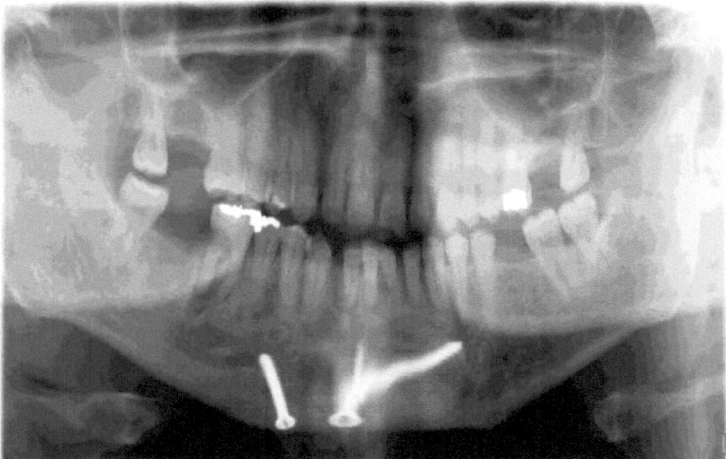

Fig. (A.8). Osteomyelitis right side of mandible after trauma.

DESCRIPTION

The right side of the body of the mandible shows signs of osteosclerosis due to an infection at the apex and furcation of the first molar. In the area of the missing second molar one can appreciate osteosclerotic bone inferior to the alveolar socket and overlapping with the inferior alveolar canal. The latter is less visible in this area. The surgical intervention probably caused the moth eaten appearance of the bone inferior to the premolars on that side.

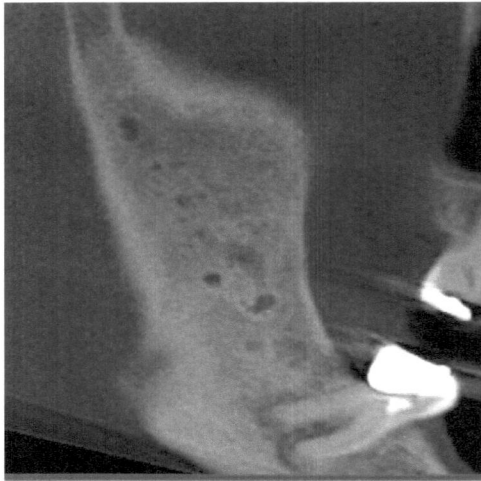

Fig. (A.9). Osteomyelitis right side of mandible.

DESCRIPTION

Notice the absence of normal trabeculation in the ramus and the angle of the mandible in this CBCT image. The apical infections on the apices of the third molar have caused the bone to react with osteosclerosis.

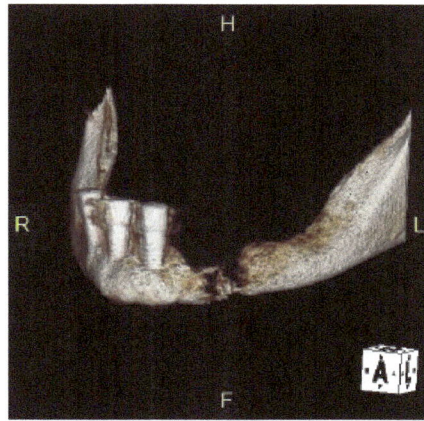

(a)

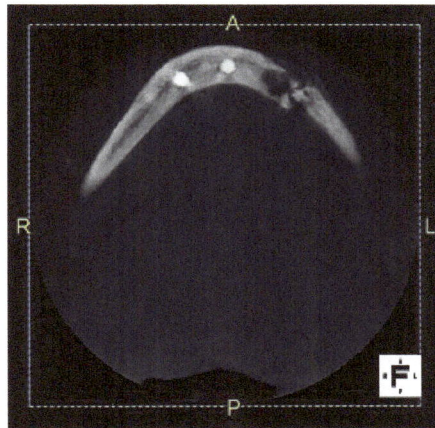

(b)

Fig. (A.10). CBCT image highlighting fracture of the mandible with associated osteomyleitis (By Màrcia F. Vasconcelos).

DESCRIPTION

The image at the top (A.10 a) is a 3D reconstructed view of CBCT while the image below is an axial view highlighting the fracture of the mandible with associated osteomyleitis. The patient was suffering from osteoporosis and was on Alendronate (Bisphosphonate) therapy. Implants were done as per treatment plan. After some months of implant placement, pain and infection appeared in the area.

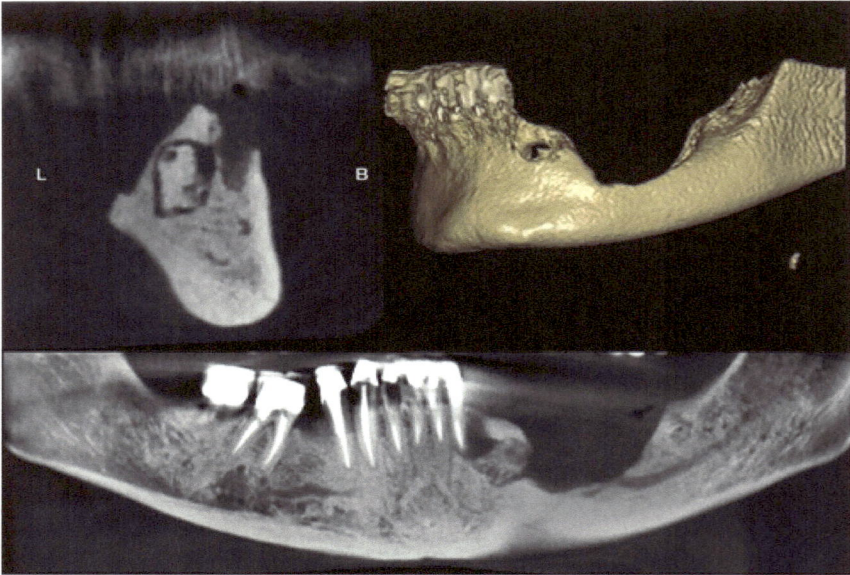

Fig. (A.11). CBCT images (sagittal, 3D reconstruction and OPG format) highlighting evidence of sequester in the left premolar region. (By Dr. Ibrahim Nasseh).

DESCRIPTION

The image at the top left is the sagittal section of the manbibular left premolar region highlighting evidence of sequesters formation. Top right image is a 3D reconstructed view of CBCT while the image below is reconstructed OPG view highlighting the osteomyelitis of left mandibular alveolus with associated sequester formation. The image also highlights the involvement of inferior alveolar canal.

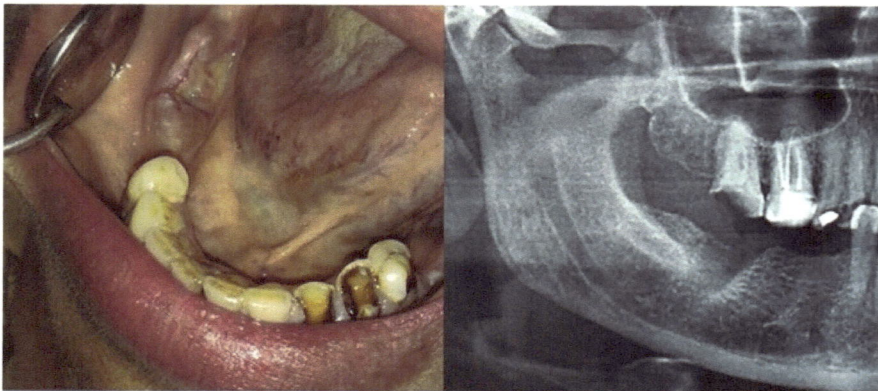

Fig. (A.12). Intraoral photograph of the patient highlighting exposed bone while cropped OPG on the right side revealing extraction socket i.r.t 47 with thickening of the trabeculae.

DESCRIPTION

The image at the left is the clinical intra oral photograph of the patient revealing exposed bone post-extraction. The image at the left is cropped OPG of the patient highlighting extraction socket in relation to 47 with evidence of thickening of the adjacent trabeculae.

Fig. (A.13). Patient presenting with extraoral sinus with pus drainage at right parasymphysis region.

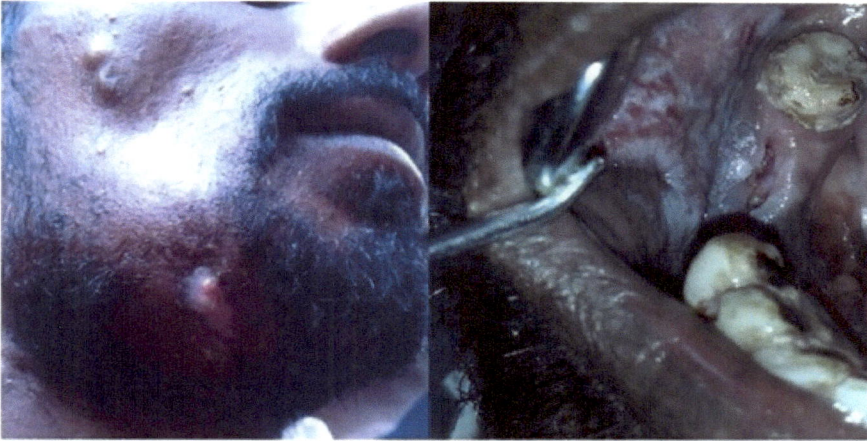

Fig. (A.13a). Extra oral and Intra oral profile with sinus and pus drainage.

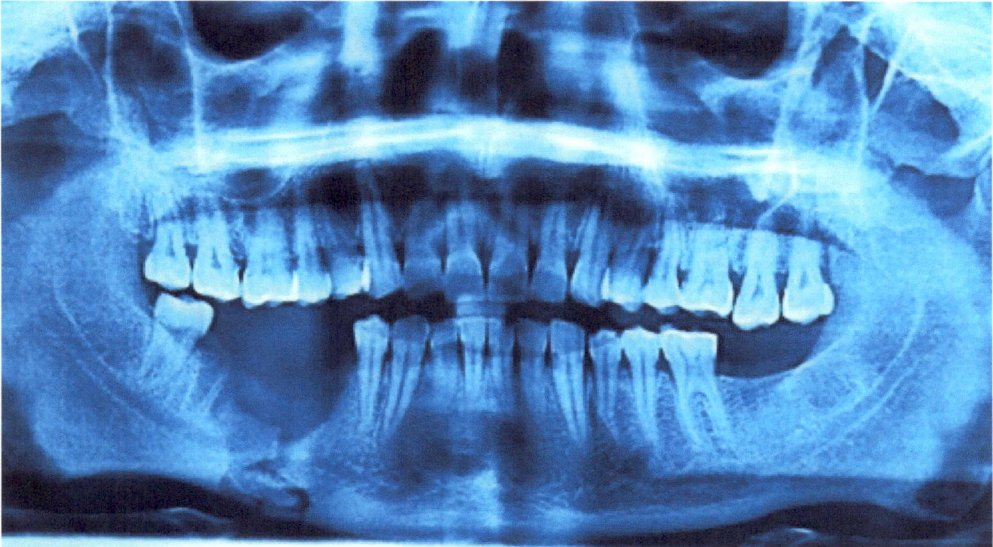

Fig. (A.13b). OPG revealing bone destruction, sequester formation and pathological fracture of the right mandibular body.

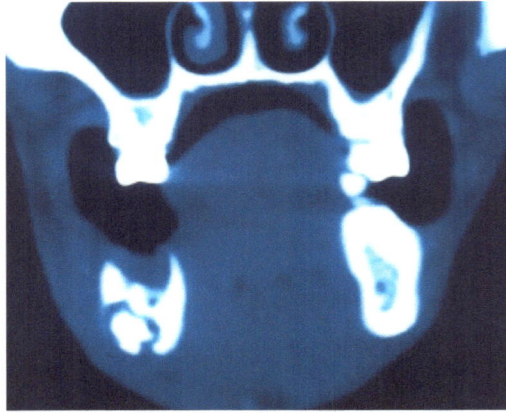

Fig. (A.13c). Coronal CT scan of the same patient revealing sequester formation in the right mandibular body.

DESCRIPTION

This patient reported to the department with an extra oral sinus and pus drainage. There was history of extraction of a carious mobile tooth in the same region few weeks back. The condition worsened and the patient presented to the department as shown in the top figure. OPG was done which revealed bone destruction in the mandibular body in relation to 45, 46, 47 with evidence of sequester formation and pathological fracture. Coronal CT section also revealed the same with a big sequester in the body. The findings suggested of the patient suffering from secondary chronic osteomyelitis or chronic suppurative osteomyelitis.

Fig. (A.14). A case of tubercular osteomyelitis of mandibular condyle.
(From Dentomaxillofacial Radiology 2012;41(2):169-74)

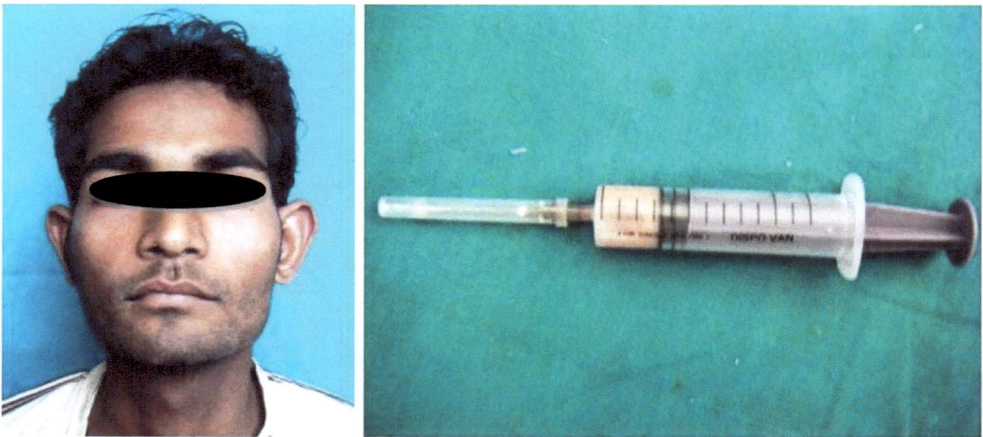

Fig. (A.14a). Patient presenting with extraoral swelling in the right preauricular region with blood tinged pus aspirated from the same.

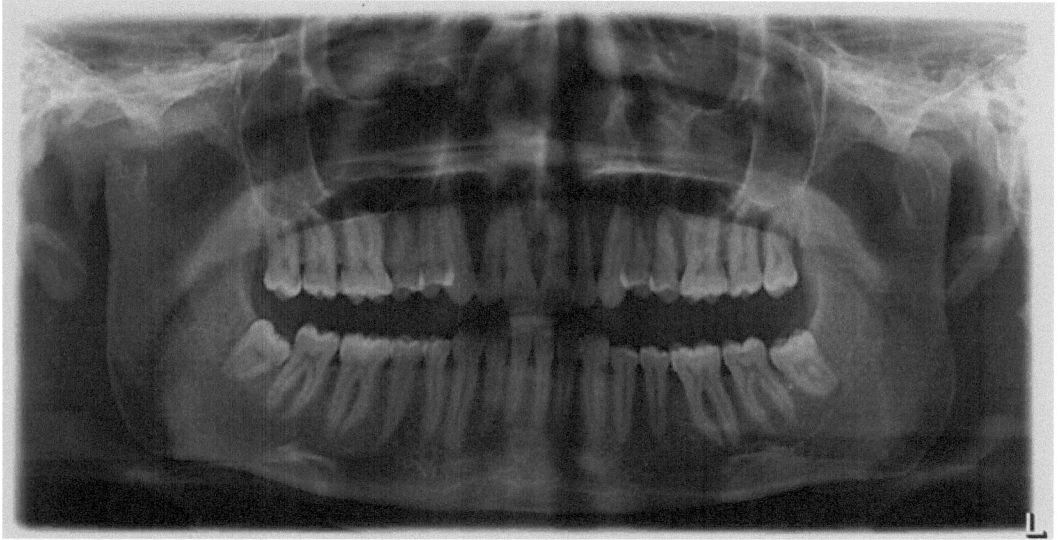

Fig. (A.14b). OPG revealing destruction of right mandibular condyle.

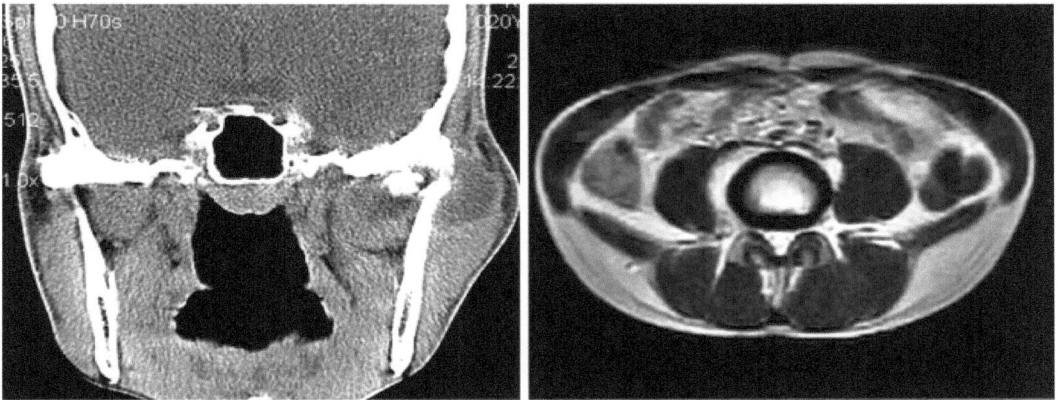

Fig. (A.14c). The left picture is Coronal CT with contrast in soft tissue winclow showing abscess surrounding the eroded right condylar process while the picture at the right reveals Axial T2W image showing bilateral paravertebral and prevertebral collections at L5-Sl.

DESCRIPTION

A 20-year-old male patient presented with a gradually progressive swelling at the right side of his face in front of the ear for about 15 days (Fig. **a**). The patient was prescribed regular antibiotics and analgesics which were of no use. The digital panoramic radiograph (Fig. **b**) revealed an ill defined area of radiolucency seen in the right mandibular condyle. CT with bone window revealed erosion with comminuted destruction of the right mandibular condyle. Soft tissue window with contrast revealed abscess formation with peripheral enhancement surrounding the right condyle (Fig. **c**). The findings correlated to Tubercular osteomyelitis of the right mandibular condyle with a surrounding abscess and cervical lymphadenopathy as the patient was suffering from TB few years back and had not taken complete medication course. Meanwhile 10 days later, the patient further complained of pain in the back. MRI was done which revealed evidence of bilateral paravertebral and pre-vertebral abscess at L5-Sl level with inflammation and erosion in the right sacroiliac joint which is highly suggestive of caries of the right sacroiliac joint. (From Dentomaxillofacial Radiology 2012;41(2):169-74).

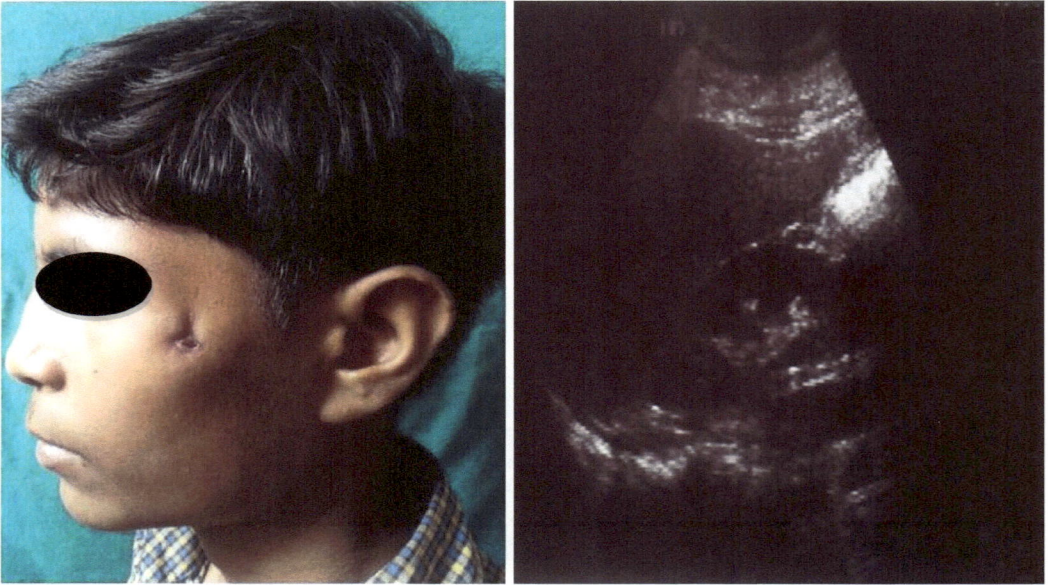

Fig. (A.15). Extraoral profile of the patient with pus draining sinus and ultrasonography with evidence of erosion and irregularity of Zygomatic bone.

DESCRIPTION

The patient presented with a chief complaint of draining pus from the left side of the cheek since 2 months. On examination, there was evidence of diffuse swelling in the left infraorbotal and zygomatic region with mild pain. The was evidence of submandibular, preauricular, post auricular and cervical lymphadenopathy. The patient was prescribed antibiotics from a local practitioner which resulted in no relief. Ultrasonography revealed erosion and irregularity of zygomatic bone of left side with small surrounding collection and internal echoes. It also revealed multiple enlarged lymph nodes in the left submandibular and left cervical region. FNAC and general physical examination by a physician confirmed Tubercular involvement.

Bibliography

[1]   Topazian RG. Osteomyelitis of the jaws In oral and maxillofacial infections. 2002; 214-239.

[2]   Nitzan DW, Marmary Y. Oateomyelitis of the mandible in a patient with osteoporosis American association of oral and maxillofacial surgeons. Page 377-380.

[3]   Asseri L, Nguvumali HI, Matee MI, Chindia ML. Chronic osteomyelitis of the mandible following tooth extraction in HIV infection. Oral Dis 1997; 3(3): 193-5.

[4]   Nordin U, Wannfors K, Colque-Navarro P, Möllby R, Heimdahl A. Antibody response in patients with osteomyelitis of the mandible. Oral Surg Oral Med Oral Pathol Oral Radiol Endod 1995; 79(4): 429-35.

[5]   Schulze D, Blessmann M, Pohlenz P, Wagner KW, Heiland M. Diagnostic criteria for the detection of mandibular osteomyelitis using cone-beam computed tomography. Dentomaxillofac Radiol 2006; 35(4): 232-5.

[6]   Lee K, Kaneda T, Mori S, Minami M, Motohashi J, Yamashiro M. Magnetic resonance imaging of normal and osteomyelitis in the mandible: assessment of short inversion time inversion recovery sequence. Oral Surg Oral Med Oral Pathol Oral Radiol Endod 2003; 96(4): 499-507.

[7]   Koorbusch GF, Fotos P, Goll KT. Retrospective assessment of osteomyelitis. Etiology, demographics, risk factors, and management in 35 cases. Oral Surg Oral Med Oral Pathol 1992; 74(2): 149-54.

[8]   Baltensperger MM, Eyrich GK, Eds. Osteomyelitis of jaws 2009.

[9]   Adekeye EO, Cornah J. Osteomyelitis of the jaws: a review of 141 cases. Br J Oral Maxillofac Surg 1985; 23(1): 24-35.

[10]   Lawoyin DO, Daramola JO, Ajagbe HA, Nyako EA, Lawoyin JO. Osteomyelitis of the mandible associated with osteopetrosis: report of a case. Br J Oral Maxillofac Surg 1988; 26(4): 330-5.

[11]   Gunge M, Yamamoto H, Katoh T, Izumi H. Suppurative osteomyelitis of the mandible in a child. Int J Oral Maxillofac Surg 1987; 16(1): 99-103.

[12]   McCash CR, Rowe NL. Acute osteomyelitis of the maxilla in infancy. J Bone Joint Surg Br 1953; 35-B(1): 22-32.

[13]   Damm N, Bouquot A. Pulpal and periapical disease Oral and Maxillofacial Pathology. 2nd edition, Saunders. An imprint of Elsevier. 2005. Pg 107-136.

[14]   Aslangul E, M'bemba J, Caillat-Vigneron N, *et al.* Diagnosing diabetic foot osteomyelitis in patients without signs of soft tissue infection by coupling hybrid ^{67}Ga SPECT/CT with bedside percutaneous bone puncture. Diabetes Care 2013; 36(8): 2203-10.

[15]   Khosla VM, Rosenfield H, Berk LH. Chronic osteomyelitis of the mandible. J Oral Surg 1971; 29(9): 649-58.

[16]   Malik NA. Osteomyelitis and Osteoradionecrosis of the jawbones, Textbook of Oral and Maxillofacial surgery, First edition 2002, Jaypee Brothers Medical Publishers Ltd, pg 593-621.

[17]   Chaudhary S, Kalra N, Gomber S. Tuberculous osteomyelitis of the mandible: a case report in a 4-year-old child. Oral Surg Oral Med Oral Pathol Oral Radiol Endod 2004; 97(5): 603-6.

[18]   Soman D, Davies SJ. A suspected case of tuberculosis of the temporomandibular joint. Br Dent J 2003; 194(1): 23-4.

[19]   Dinkar AD, Prabhudessai V. Primary tuberculous osteomyelitis of the mandible: a case report. Dentomaxillofac Radiol 2008; 37(7): 415-20.

[20]   Wannfors K, Gazelius B. Blood flow in jaw bones affected by chronic osteomyelitis. Br J Oral

Maxillofac Surg 1991; 29(3): 147-53.

[21]   Eyrich GK, Baltensperger MM, Bruder E, Graetz KW. Primary chronic osteomyelitis in childhood and adolescence: a retrospective analysis of 11 cases and review of the literature. J Oral Maxillofac Surg 2003; 61(5): 561-73.

[22]   Suei Y, Taguchi A, Tanimoto K. Diagnosis and classification of mandibular osteomyelitis. Oral Surg Oral Med Oral Pathol Oral Radiol Endod 2005; 100(2): 207-14.

[23]   Parker ME. Infections of the teeth and jaws. Oral Maxill Diagn Imag 1993; 181-209.

[24]   Suei Y, Taguchi A, Tanimoto K. Diffuse sclerosing osteomyelitis of the mandible: its characteristics and possible relationship to synovitis, acne, pustulosis, hyperostosis, osteitis (SAPHO) syndrome. J Oral Maxillofac Surg 1996; 54(10): 1194-9.

[25]   Tanaka R, Hayashi T. Computed tomography findings of chronic osteomyelitis involving the mandible: correlation to histopathological findings. Dentomaxillofac Radiol 2008; 37(2): 94-103.

[26]   Aliabadi P, Nikpoor N. Imaging Osteomyelitis Arthritis and Rheumstism 1994; 37: 617-22.

[27]   Yoshiura K, Hijiya T, Ariji E, *et al.* Radiographic patterns of osteomyelitis in the mandible. Plain film/CT correlation. Oral Surg Oral Med Oral Pathol 1994; 78(1): 116-24.

[28]   Worth HM, Stoneman DW. Osteomyelitis, malignant disease, and fibrous dysplasia. Some radiologic similarities and differences. Dent Radiogr Photogr 1977; 50(1): 1-8, 12-15.

[29]   Taori KB, Solanke R, Mahajan SM, Rangankar V, Saini TC. Evaluation of mandibular osteomyelitis. Ind J Radiol Imag 2005; 154: 447-51.

[30]   Coviello V, Stevens MR. Contemporary concepts in the treatment of chronic osteomyelitis. Oral Maxillofac Surg Clin North Am 2007; 19(4): 523-534, vi.

[31]   Kashima I, Tajima K, Nishimura K, *et al.* Diagnostic imaging of diseases affecting the mandible with the use of computed panoramic radiography. Oral Surg Oral Med Oral Pathol 1990; 70(1): 110-6.

[32]   Tang JS, Gold RH, Bassett LW, Seeger LL. Musculoskeletal infection of the extremities: evaluation with MR imaging. Radiology 1988; 166(1 Pt 1): 205-9.

[33]   Schmidt ER, Townsend J. Unusual complication of subacute osteomyelitis following tibial bone graft: report of a case. J Oral Maxillofac Surg 2008; 66(6): 1290-3.

[34]   Lee L. Inflammatory lesions of the jaws.Oral radiology: principles and intertpretation 5th ed. 5th ed.2004; 366-83.

[35]   Chukwudum U, Robert M, Amy C, Daniel T, DeSimone J. Osteomyelitis Of The Jaw: A Retrospective Analysis. Int J Infect Dis 2009; 7(2): 13.

[36]   Johnston B, Conly J. Osteomyelitis management: More art than science? Can J Infect Dis Med Microbiol 2007; 18(2): 115-8.

[37]   Mader JT, Shirtliff M, Calhoun JH. Staging and staging application in osteomyelitis. Clin Infect Dis 1997; 25(6): 1303-9.

[38]   Pineda C, Espinosa R, Pena A. Radiographic imaging in osteomyelitis: the role of plain radiography, computed tomography, ultrasonography, magnetic resonance imaging, and scintigraphy. Semin Plast Surg 2009; 23(2): 80-9.

[39]   Gold RH, Hawkins RA, Katz RD. Bacterial osteomyelitis: findings on plain radiography, CT, MR, and scintigraphy. AJR Am J Roentgenol 1991; 157(2): 365-70.

[40]   Cierny G III, Mader JT, Penninck JJ. A clinical staging system for adult osteomyelitis. Clin Orthop Relat Res 2003; (414): 7-24.

[41]   Bohndorf K. Infection of the appendicular skeleton. Eur Radiol 2004; 14 (Suppl. 3): E53-63.

[42]   Fritz JM, McDonald JR. Osteomyelitis: approach to diagnosis and treatment. Phys Sportsmed 2008;

36(1): a116823.

[43]   Schwegler B, Stumpe KD, Weishaupt D, *et al.* Unsuspected osteomyelitis is frequent in persistent diabetic foot ulcer and better diagnosed by MRI than by 18F-FDG PET or 99mTc-MOAB. J Intern Med 2008; 263(1): 99-106.

[44]   Meyers SP, Wiener SN. Diagnosis of hematogenous pyogenic vertebral osteomyelitis by magnetic resonance imaging. Arch Intern Med 1991; 151(4): 683-7.

[45]   Kocher MS, Lee B, Dolan M, Weinberg J, Shulman ST. Pediatric orthopedic infections: early detection and treatment. Pediatr Ann 2006; 35(2): 112-22.

[46]   Hui CL, Naidoo P. Extramedullary fat fluid level on MRI as a specific sign for osteomyelitis. Australas Radiol 2003; 47(4): 443-6.

[47]   Littenberg B, Mushlin AI. Technetium bone scanning in the diagnosis of osteomyelitis: a meta-analysis of test performance. J Gen Intern Med 1992; 7(2): 158-64.

[48]   Collado P, Naredo E, Calvo C, Crespo M. Role of power Doppler sonography in early diagnosis of osteomyelitis in children. J Clin Ultrasound 2008; 36(4): 251-3.

[49]   Kaiser S, Rosenborg M. Early detection of subperiosteal abscesses by ultrasonography. A means for further successful treatment in pediatric osteomyelitis. Pediatr Radiol 1994; 24(5): 336-9.

[50]   Sivapathasundharam: Diseases of the pulp and periapical tissues Shafer's textbook of oral pathology 5th ed. 5th ed.2006; 659-96.

[51]   Ghom Anil Govindarao. Infections Of The Oral Cavity & Oral Sepsis, Textbook of oral medicine, First Edition 2005 Jaypee Medical Publishers P Ltd. pg381- 439.

[52]   Mercuri LG. Acute Osteomyelitis of the jaws. Oral Maxil Surg Clin 1991; 3: 355.

[53]   Linda L. Inflammatory lesions of the jaws 2000.

[54]   Saraswathi TR, Ranganathan K, Balasundaram S, Kirankumar K. Osteomyelitis of the jaws: A Review. J Oral Maxillofac Pathol 2002; 6(2): 1-9.

[55]   Bitting ND, Durham NC. Acute osteomyelitis and complications. South Med J 1929; 22(6): 580-3.

[56]   Caldwell R. Acute Osteomyelitis. South Med J 1909; 1163-6.

[57]   Goodwin WH. Osteomyelitis. South Med J 1939; 27(7): 583-90.

[58]   Fenner ED. Acute Osteomyelitis. South Med J 1932; 25(4): 355-7.

[59]   Oechsner JF. Acute Suppurative Osteomyelitis. South Med J 1915; 678-80.

[60]   Sheikh S, Pallagatti S, Aggarwal A, Gupta D, Puri N, Mittal A. Osteosarcoma of maxilla: A case report. J Clin Exp Dent 2010; 2(3): e117-20.

[61]   Petrikowski CG, Pharoah MJ, Lee L, Grace MG. Radiographic differentiation of osteogenic sarcoma, osteomyelitis, and fibrous dysplasia of the jaws. Oral Surg Oral Med Oral Pathol Oral Radiol Endod 1995; 80(6): 744-50.

[62]   Schuknecht BF, Carls FR, Valavanis A, Sailer HF. Mandibular osteomyelitis: evaluation and staging in 18 patients, using magnetic resonance imaging, computed tomography and conventional radiographs. J Craniomaxillofac Surg 1997; 25(1): 24-33.

[63]   Harris LF. Chronic mandibular osteomyelitis. South Med J 1986; 79(6): 696-7.

[64]   Klinefelter ML. Osteomyelitis. South Med J 1929; 19(5): 347-50.

[65]   Taori KB, Mahajan SM, Rangankar V, *et al.* CT evaluation of mandibular osteomyelitis. Ind J Radiol Imag 2005; 15: 447-51.

[66]   Montonen M, Iizuka T, Hallikainen D, Lindqvist C. Decortication in the treatment of diffuse sclerosing osteomyelitis of the mandible. Retrospective analysis of 41 cases between 1969 and 1990.

Oral Surg Oral Med Oral Pathol 1993; 75(1): 5-11.

[67]   Baltensperger M, Grätz K, Bruder E, Lebeda R, Makek M, Eyrich G. Is primary chronic osteomyelitis a uniform disease? Proposal of a classification based on a retrospective analysis of patients treated in the past 30 years. J Craniomaxillofac Surg 2004; 32(1): 43-50.

[68]   Bevin CR, Inwards CY, Keller EE. Surgical management of primary chronic osteomyelitis: a long-term retrospective analysis. J Oral Maxillofac Surg 2008; 66(10): 2073-85.

[69]   Frid P, Tornes K, Nielsen Ø, Skaug N. Primary chronic osteomyelitis of the jaw--a microbial investigation using cultivation and DNA analysis: a pilot study. Oral Surg Oral Med Oral Pathol Oral Radiol Endod 2009; 107(5): 641-7.

[70]   Kahn MF, Hayem F, Hayem G, Grossin M. Is diffuse sclerosing osteomyelitis of the mandible part of the synovitis, acne, pustulosis, hyperostosis, osteitis (SAPHO) syndrome? Analysis of seven cases. Oral Surg Oral Med Oral Pathol 1994; 78(5): 594-8.

[71]   Marx RE, Carlson ER, Smith BR, Toraya N. Isolation of Actinomyces species and Eikenella corrodens from patients with chronic diffuse sclerosing osteomyelitis. J Oral Maxillofac Surg 1994; 52(1): 26-33.

[72]   Suei Y, Taguchi A, Tanimoto K. Diagnostic points and possible origin of osteomyelitis in synovitis, acne, pustulosis, hyperostosis and osteitis (SAPHO) syndrome: a radiographic study of 77 mandibular osteomyelitis cases. Rheumatology (Oxford) 2003; 42(11): 1398-403.

[73]   Otsuka K, Hamakawa H, Kayahara H, Tanioka H. Chronic recurrent multifocal osteomyelitis involving the mandible in a 4-year-old girl: a case report and a review of the literature. J Oral Maxillofac Surg 1999; 57(8): 1013-6.

[74]   Flygare L, Norderyd J, Kubista J, Ohlsson J, Vallo-Christiansen J, Magnusson B. Chronic recurrent multifocal osteomyelitis involving both jaws: report of a case including magnetic resonance correlation. Oral Surg Oral Med Oral Pathol Oral Radiol Endod 1997; 83(2): 300-5.

[75]   Suei Y, Tanimoto K, Taguchi A, Wada T, Ishikawa T. Chronic recurrent multifocal osteomyelitis involving the mandible. Oral Surg Oral Med Oral Pathol 1994; 78(2): 156-62.

[76]   Suei Y, Tanimoto K, Taguchi A, *et al.* Possible identity of diffuse sclerosing osteomyelitis and chronic recurrent multifocal osteomyelitis. One entity or two. Oral Surg Oral Med Oral Pathol Oral Radiol Endod 1995; 80(4): 401-8.

[77]   Cyrlak D, Pais MJ. Chronic recurrent multifocal osteomyelitis. Skeletal Radiol 1986; 15(1): 32-9.

[78]   Mortensson W, Edeburn G, Fries M, Nilsson R. Chronic recurrent multifocal osteomyelitis in children. A roentgenologic and scintigraphic investigation. Acta Radiol 1988; 29(5): 565-70.

[79]   Bjorksten B, Boquist L. Histological aspects of Chronic recurrent multifocal osteomyelitis. J Bone Joint Surg Br 1980; 62: 376-80.

[80]   Donohue WB, Abelardo LM. Osteomyelitis of the jaw. Can Med Assoc J 1970; 103(7): 748-50.

[81]   Fullmer JM, Scarfe WC, Kushner GM, Alpert B, Farman AG. Cone beam computed tomographic findings in refractory chronic suppurative osteomyelitis of the mandible. Br J Oral Maxillofac Surg 2007; 45(5): 364-71.

[82]   Calhoun KH, Shapiro RD, Stiernberg CM, Calhoun JH, Mader JT. Osteomyelitis of the mandible. Arch Otolaryngol Head Neck Surg 1988; 114(10): 1157-62.

[83]   Dabney MY, Dabney EB, Loranz CP. A new treatment for osteomyelitis. South Med J 1934; 27(4): 372-3.

[84]   McKeever DC. The classic: maggots in treatment of osteomyelitis: a simple inexpensive method. 1933. Clin Orthop Relat Res 2008; 466(6): 1329-35.

[85]   Baer WS. The Treatment of Chronic Osteomyelitis with the Maggot (Larva of the Blow Fly). J Bone Joint Surg Br 1931; 13: 438.

[86]   Livingston SK, Prince LH. The Treatment of Chronic Osteomyelitis with Special Reference to the Use of the Maggot Active Principle. J Am Med Assn 1932; 98: 1143.

[87]   Fang RC, Galiano RD. Adjunctive therapies in the treatment of osteomyelitis. Semin Plast Surg 2009; 23(2): 141-7.

[88]   Lentrodt S, Lentrodt J, Kübler N, Mödder U. Hyperbaric oxygen for adjuvant therapy for chronically recurrent mandibular osteomyelitis in childhood and adolescence. J Oral Maxillofac Surg 2007; 65(2): 186-91.

[89]   Jacoby NM, Sagorin L. Osteomyelitis Of The Jaws In Infancy Treated With Penicillin. Archives Of Disease In Chi Arch Dis Child 1945; 20: 166-8.

[90]   Goldbloom A, Bacal HL. Osteomyelitis Of The Superior Maxilla In New-Born Infants. Can Med Assoc J 1937; 37(5): 443-5.

[91]   Dunphy DL, Frazer JP. Acute osteomyelitis of the maxilla in a newborn; report of a case successfully treated with penicillin and sulfadiazine. Yale J Biol Med 1947; 19(5): 877-81.

[92]   Wilensky AO. The pathogenesis and treatment of acute osteomyelitis of the jaws in nurslings and in infants. Am J Dis Child 1932; 43: 431.

[93]   Wilensky AO. Osteomyelitis of the Jaws in Nurslings and Infants. Ann Surg 1932; 95(1): 33-45.

[94]   Johnston B, Conly J. Osteomyelitis management: More art than science? Can J Infect Dis Med Microbiol 2007; 18(2): 115-8.

[95]   Euba G, Murillo O, Fernández-Sabé N, *et al.* Long-term follow-up trial of oral rifampin-cotrimoxazole combination versus intravenous cloxacillin in treatment of chronic staphylococcal osteomyelitis. Antimicrob Agents Chemother 2009; 53(6): 2672-6.

[96]   Lazzarini L, Lipsky BA, Mader JT. Antibiotic treatment of osteomyelitis: what have we learned from 30 years of clinical trials? Int J Infect Dis 2005; 9: 127-38.

[97]   Wong JK, Wood RE, McLean M. Conservative management of osteoradionecrosis. Oral Surg Oral Med Oral Pathol Oral Radiol Endod 1997; 84(1): 16-21.

[98]   van Merkesteyn JP, Balm AJ, Bakker DJ, Borgmeyer-Hoelen AM. Hyperbaric oxygen treatment of osteoradionecrosis of the mandible with repeated pathologic fracture. Report of a case. Oral Surg Oral Med Oral Pathol 1994; 77(5): 461-4.

[99]   Marx RE, Johnson RP, Kline SN. Prevention of osteoradionecrosis: a randomized prospective clinical trial of hyperbaric oxygen versus penicillin. J Am Dent Assoc 1985; 111(1): 49-54.

[100] Hewitt C, Farah CS. Bisphosphonate-related osteonecrosis of the jaws: a comprehensive review. J Oral Pathol Med 2007; 36(6): 319-28.

[101] Brooks JK, Gilson AJ, Sindler AJ, Ashman SG, Schwartz KG, Nikitakis NG. Osteonecrosis of the jaws associated with use of risedronate: report of 2 new cases. Oral Surg Oral Med Oral Pathol Oral Radiol Endod 2007; 103(6): 780-6.

[102] Ruggiero SL, Mehrotra B, Rosenberg TJ, Engroff SL. Osteonecrosis of the jaws associated with the use of bisphosphonates: a review of 63 cases. J Oral Maxillofac Surg 2004; 62(5): 527-34.

[103] Chiandussi S, Biasotto M, Dore F, Cavalli F, Cova MA, Di Lenarda R. Clinical and diagnostic imaging of bisphosphonate-associated osteonecrosis of the jaws. Dentomaxillofac Radiol 2006; 35(4): 236-43.

[104] Ahmed I, Abbas SZ, Haque F, Rashid M, Ahmed SA. "Osteomyelitis of mandible"- A rare presentation of osteopetrosis. Ind J Radiol Imag 2006; 16(2): 253-6.

[105] Oğütcen-Toller M, Tek M, Sener I, Bereket C, I'nal S, Özden B. Intractable bimaxillary osteomyelitis in osteopetrosis: review of the literature and current therapy. J Oral Maxillofac Surg 2010; 68(1): 167-75.

[106] Uche C, Mogyoros R, Chang A, Taub D, DeSimone J. Osteomyelitis Of The Jaw: A Retrospective Analysis. Int J Infect Dis 2009; 7(2): 1-7.

[107] Olaitan AA, Amuda JT, Adekeye EO. Osteomyelitis of the mandible in sickle cell disease. Br J Oral Maxillofac Surg 1997; 35(3): 190-2.

[108] Soubrier M, Dubost JJ, Ristori JM, Sauvezie B, Bussière JL. Pamidronate in the treatment of diffuse sclerosing osteomyelitis of the mandible. Oral Surg Oral Med Oral Pathol Oral Radiol Endod 2001; 92(6): 637-40.

[109] García-Marín F, Iriarte-Ortabe JI, Reychler H. Chronic diffuse sclerosing osteomyelitis of the mandible or mandibular location of S.A.P.H.O. syndrome. Acta Stomatol Belg 1996; 93(2): 65-71.

[110] Montonen M, Kalso E, Pylkkären L, Lindströrm BM, Lindqvist C. Disodium clodronate in the treatment of diffuse sclerosing osteomyelitis (DSO) of the mandible. Int J Oral Maxillofac Surg 2001; 30(4): 313-7.

[111] Van Merkesteyn JP, Groot RH, Bras J, *et al.* DSO of the mandible: a new concept of its etiology. Oral Surg Oral Med Oral Pathol 1990; 70: 414-9.

[112] Ogawa A, Miyate H, Nakamura Y, Shimada M, Seki S, Kudo K. Treating chronic diffuse sclerosing osteomyelitis of the mandible with saucerization and autogenous bone grafting. Oral Surg Oral Med Oral Pathol Oral Radiol Endod 2001; 91(4): 390-4.

[113] Suei Y, Tanimoto K, Miyauchi M, Ishikawa T. Partial resection of the mandible for the treatment of diffuse sclerosing osteomyelitis: Report of four cases. J Oral Maxil Surg 1997; 55: 410-4; 414-5.

[114] Migliorati CA, Schubert MM, Peterson DE, Seneda LM. Bisphosphonate-associated osteonecrosis of mandibular and maxillary bone: an emerging oral complication of supportive cancer therapy. Cancer 2005; 104(1): 83-93.

[115] Jacobsson S. Diffuse sclerosing osteomyelitis of the mandible. Int J Oral Surg 1984; 13(5): 363-85.

[116] Martin-Granizo R, Garcia-Gonzalez D, Sastre J, Diaz FJ. Mandibular sclerosing osteomyelitis of Garré. Otolaryngol Head Neck Surg 1999; 121(6): 828-9.

[117] Suma R, Vinay C, Shashikanth MC, Subba Reddy VV. Garre's sclerosing osteomyelitis. J Indian Soc Pedod Prev Dent 2007; 25 (Suppl.): S30-3.

[118] Norden CW. Lessons learned from animal models of osteomyelitis. Rev Infect Dis 1988; 10(1): 103-10.

[119] Waldvogel FA. Osteomyelitis. In: Gorbach SL, Bartlett JG, Blacklow NR, editors. Infectious Diseases. Philadelphia: Saunders; 1988: 1339-44.

[120] Dworkin R, Modin G, Kunz S, Rich R, Zak O, Sande M. Comparative efficacies of ciprofloxacin, pefloxacin, and vancomycin in combination with rifampin in a rat model of methicillin-resistant *Staphylococcus aureus* chronic osteomyelitis. Antimicrob Agents Chemother 1990; 34(6): 1014-6.

[121] Norden CW. Experimental chronic staphylococcal osteomyelitis in rabbits: treatment with rifampin alone and in combination with other antimicrobial agents. Rev Infect Dis 1983; 5 (Suppl. 3): S491-4.

[122] Mader JT, Adams K, Morrison L. Comparative evaluation of cefazolin and clindamycin in the treatment of experimental *Staphylococcus aureus* osteomyelitis in rabbits. Antimicrob Agents Chemother 1989; 33(10): 1760-4.

[123] Ang JY, Asmar BI. Multidrug-resistant viridans streptococcus (MDRVS) osteomyelitis of the mandible successfully treated with moxifloxacin. South Med J 2008; 101(5): 539-40.

[124] Nelson CL, McLaren SG, Skinner RA, Smeltzer MS, Thomas JR, Olsen KM. The treatment of experimental osteomyelitis by surgical debridement and the implantation of calcium sulfate tobramycin pellets. J Orthop Res 2002; 20(4): 643-7.

[125] Holly D, Jurkovic R, Mracna J. Condensing osteitis in oral region. Bratisl Lek Listy (Tlacene Vyd)

2009; 110(11): 713-5.

[126] Sheikh S, Pallagatti S, Gupta D, Mittal A. Tuberculous osteomyelitis of mandibular condyle: a diagnostic dilemma. Dentomaxillofac Radiol 2012; 41(2): 169-74.

[127] Gupta D, Sheikh S, Pallagatti S, Aggarwal A, Singh R, Mittal A. Osteomyelitis of the mandible mimicking fibrous dysplasia: A radiographic controversy. Clin Dent 2013; 7(3): 20-5.

[128] Sheikh S, Pallagatti S, Gupta D, Aggarwal A, Singh R, Sharma R. Chronic Suppurative Osteomyelitis of Maxilla: A Case Report. EC Dental Science 2015; 1(3): 126-31.

[129] Gupta D. Oro-Maxillofacial Radiology and Imaging: An Indispensable Dental Specialty. The Open Dent J 2015; 9(Suppl 2: M1): 260-2.

[130] Gupta D. Role of Maxillofacial Radiology and Imaging in the diagnosis and Treatment of Osteomyelitis of the Jaws. J Dent Oral Disord Ther 2015; 3(2): 1-2.

[131] Gupta D. Oro-Maxillofacial Radiology and Imaging: An update. Open Dent J 2017; 9(Suppl 3: M1)

SUBJECT INDEX

A

Activity 38, 39, 40
  increased bone turnover 38
  normal osteoblastic bone 40
  osteoblastic 39, 40
Acute osteomyelitis (AO) 3, 16, 21, 22, 24, 25,
  26, 29, 32, 37, 38, 39, 43, 45, 46, 47, 49,
  50, 51, 52, 53, 54, 57, 58, 61, 76, 79, 80,
  82, 83, 84, 98, 99, 109, 116
Acute suppurative osteomyelitis 22, 45, 47
Adult-onset primary chronic osteomyelitis 64,
  65
Albers–Schonberg disease 87, 88
Albuminuria 49, 50
Alveolar osteitis 26
Anaemia 5, 6, 8, 90
Anaerobic osteomyelitis 81
Anatomical disease types 17
Anorexia 48, 49, 56
Antibiotics 3, 4, 5, 6, 56, 69, 76, 78, 80, 82,
  84, 86, 89, 90, 91, 92, 93, 96, 97, 98, 99,
  100, 101, 103, 108, 109, 117, 118
  spectrum 82, 89, 90
  systemic 98, 103
Antibiotic therapy 2, 5, 17, 22, 23, 74, 75, 80,
  83, 85, 86, 90, 95, 98, 99, 100, 110, 118
  prolonged 90, 110
Antibiotic treatment 63, 92, 99, 100
Anti-inflammatory drugs 24, 92, 93, 94, 97, 98
Asymptomatic cases 114
Autologous corticocancellous bone grafts 112

B

Bacteria, infecting 77
Bacterial infection 24, 63, 88, 95
  secondary 88
Bacterial osteomyelitis 23, 24
Bisphosphonates 87, 88, 92, 93, 94
Blood cells, white 10, 89
Blood flow 44, 94

Blood supply 2, 13, 14, 92, 111
Bone 1, 2, 3, 5, 8, 9, 10, 11, 12, 13, 14, 15, 16,
  17, 18, 26, 29, 30, 31, 32, 33, 35, 37, 39,
  40, 42, 45, 47, 48, 50, 51, 52, 53, 56, 58,
  60, 67, 69, 70, 71, 73, 74, 77, 78, 79, 80,
  81, 82, 84, 86, 87, 88, 89, 92, 95, 96, 99,
  100, 101, 102, 103, 104, 105, 108, 109,
  110, 111, 112, 113, 114, 115, 116, 117
  adjacent 45
  alveolar 26
  bleeding 103, 109
  cancellous 14, 17, 30, 35, 37, 81, 112
  compact 37
  dense 114
  healthy 8, 10
  hyoid 32
  hypocellular 89
  infected 40, 79, 100, 103, 117
  irradiated 86
  limb 74
  malar 9
  medullary 17
  multiple 69
  necrotic 12, 52, 77, 88, 100
  radiopaque 52
  reconstructed 92
  residual 102
  spongy 74
Bone alteration 29
Bone aspirate 72
Bone biopsy 71
Bone conditions, pathological 40
Bone destruction 29, 30, 37, 38, 51, 52, 54,
  113
  focal 37
  ill-defined 54
  showed permeative 38
Bone dissolution 29
Bone enlargement 68
Bone formation 52, 54, 62, 96
  reactive 52, 54, 62
  reactive peripheral 96

www.ingramcontent.com/pod-product-compliance
Lightning Source LLC
Chambersburg PA
CBHW041711210326
41598CB00007B/615